The
Lazy Girl's Guide
to **Good Sex**

Anita Naik is a freelance writer, author and columnist. She specialises in health, sex and lifestyle issues and writes for *Red*, *Now*, *Zest* and *Closer* and is the resident agony aunt on *TV Quick* magazine. She is also the author of over 30 books and was previously the agony aunt on *Just17* and *Closer* magazine, and the sex columnist on *More!*.

Anita is also the author of:

The Lazy Girl's Guide to Beauty

The Lazy Girl's Guide to Good Health

The Lazy Girl's Guide to a Fabulous Body

The Lazy Girl's Party Guide

The Lazy Girl's Guide to Men

Babe Bible

The New You

Pocket Babe

The
Lazy Girl's Guide
to **Good Sex**

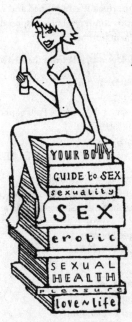

Anita Naik

PIATKUS

PIATKUS

First published in Great Britain in 2002 by Piatkus Books
Copyright © 2002 Anita Naik
Reprinted 2002, 2003, 2004, 2006, 2007
This edition published in 2008
The moral right of the authors has been asserted

A CIP catalogue record for this book is available from the British Library

ISBN 978-0-7499-4161-1

Designed and typeset in Minion and Avenir by Paul Saunders
Edited by Jan Cutler
Cover and inside illustrations by Nicola Cramp
Printed in the UK by CPI Mackays, Chatham, ME5 8TD

Papers used by Piatkus Books are natural, renewable and recyclable
products made from wood grown in sustainable forests and certified
in accordance with the rules of the Forest Stewardship Council.

Mixed Sources
Product group from well-managed
forests and other controlled sources
www.fsc.org Cert no. SGS-COC-004081
FSC © 1996 Forest Stewardship Council

Piatkus Books
An imprint of
Little, Brown Book Group
100 Victoria Embankment
London EC4Y ODY

An Hachette Livre UK Company
www.hachettelivre.co.uk

www.piatkus.co.uk

Contents

Acknowledgements   vi

Introduction   1

1   The basic stuff   5

2   The solo stuff   32

3   The sex stuff   57

4   The orgasm stuff   89

5   The problematic stuff   114

6   The kinky stuff   135

7   The sensible stuff   160

8   How to be extremely knowledgeable about sex (without trying)   191

Resources: help, advice, information and naughty shopping   205

Index   210

Acknowledgements

Thanks to all the lazy girls who willingly gave me their lazy sex tips but paid me huge amounts to keep their names out of the book. You know who you are!

Introduction

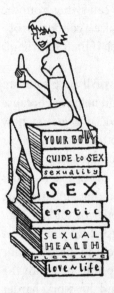

Why this book can help you

Sex – everyone's doing it. Right? Well, if studies are to be believed not only are less of us bothering to tear up the sheets every night but most of us can't even be bothered to give it 100 per cent when we do. Little wonder then that common complaints about adventures in the bedroom include gripes about lazy lovers, sexual boredom and the inevitable no-show orgasms.

However, lazy sex isn't just about being too lazy to do it. It's about being too lazy to find new ways of adding creativity, energy and fun to your sex life. It's about putting up with lazy lovers because you're too embarrassed to say anything or do anything, and, more importantly, it's about sex that is dominated by the myths and assumptions you've been carrying around with you since you were 13 years old. Beliefs, for example, that women have lower sex drives than men, sex is only exciting in the beginning, and the notoriously infamous – men are up for it any time and with anyone. If you're currently having sex in any of the above ways, or if sex makes you wonder why you're even bothering to take your clothes off, you're having lazy sex.

The good news is you're not alone – take it from me, I read over 2,000 letters a year from people with sexual problems! The truth is most of us (despite what we'll admit to in public) have had our fair share of sexual embarrassments, disasters and hiccups mostly caused by useless lovers, lack of knowledge and limited experience. I know girls who have had men fall asleep on them mid-act, friends who can swing from the rafters during sex but don't know how to use a condom properly and guys who find it impossible to tell if their girlfriends have ever had an orgasm.

If any of the above sound familiar, you'll be pleased to know *The Lazy Girl's Guide to Good Sex* can help you, because whether you're spectacularly lazy in bed, at a loss at how to change your sexual patterns for the better or simply eager for more sexual tips and advice, the answers are in the following pages. The best part is that unlike other sex manuals you won't have to search for these tips among embarrassing legs-wide-open shots, readers' wives scenarios and/or gory porn-film language. Plus I won't be suggesting you peer at your genitalia with a mirror, telling you to perfect your demanding dominatrix side and/or jump into bed with the first attractive man you see and demand he work harder (though this can work).

Instead this book is about how you can have good sex whenever you want. Sex that leaves you feeling sexy, fulfilled and at ease with your body. This is why we're first going back to those early teenage fumbles and moving right through to where you are today and beyond. If you're still asking yourself: 'What's the point of reading about sex, because the act of sex is obvious', ponder this:

The secret to having good sex is about more than knowing the right moves or saying the right things in bed. It's about expanding your sexual knowledge and in doing so learning to get exactly what you need from sex. Perfect your technique and you'll not only boost your enjoyment but also that of your partners. So, even if you are too lazy at heart to go at it for longer than five minutes, they'll still be five minutes well worth bragging about.

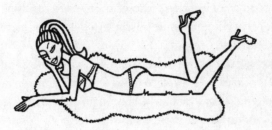

CHAPTER ONE

The basic stuff

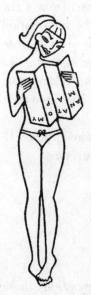

ARE YOU GOOD IN BED? Is your mind a limitless vault of intriguing sexual positions? Can you orgasm at the drop of a hat, satisfy your partner, satiate yourself and still find the energy to go at it ten times a night? If you can, congratulations. However, if you happen to be a girl who fakes it more times than she makes it, it's time to ditch the self-limiting beliefs and take some tips on how to spice up your sex life.

The good news is anyone, even the laziest girl, can boost her sexual satisfaction by simply arming herself with the right kind of information. This means relearning those biology basics, going right back to the beginning and then moving forward from there. Do it right and you'll not only become an ace at level-one sexual manoeuvres but you'll have more orgasms, partners who beg you for more and a thriving and frisky sexual mind.

The biology basics

Sex surveys show that most of us know hardly anything about our sexual anatomy. In fact in one major US university study four out of ten men didn't know where the clitoris was, and six out of ten had never even heard of the female G-spot. Women didn't fare much better with three out of ten having no idea what the male G-spot was and six out of ten mixing up the scrotum with the testicles.

Laugh you may but the fact remains, apart from a few school biology lessons on the facts of life, the information most of us know about sexual anatomy tends to come from our sexual experience. This is great if you've had an A-list teacher but not so fabulous if you've had a series of lazy lovers who have been happy to let you fumble your way round their lazy bods.

So for those who need a quick body rundown here's all you'll ever need to know about the body's sexual bits.

Your anatomy map

The breasts

Small, large, lopsided, pert, droopy or flat – breasts are those spherical objects you hoist daily into your bra. On a simple anatomical level, breasts are simply fatty tissue with the only muscle in the whole area being the nipple. However, on the sexual front you don't need me to tell you that the breasts, nipples and areola (pigmented area surrounding the nipple) are hugely sexually responsive to touch. Which is why the whole area swells during sexual arousal.

The nipple is the most sensitive area of the breast as it's made up of erectile tissue and super nerves, which means the whole area enlarges and becomes sexually sensitive when stimulated by touch or the cold.

Do feel your breasts to discover how you like them to be touched and felt.

Don't allow your lovers to be nipple-obsessed. The nipple likes to be pawed but not if the rest of the breast is being neglected.

Vulva

Not a posh Scandinavian car but a name you probably never use, and why would you? The vulva is one of those anatomically correct terms that only doctors use to describe the external sex organs. Basically speaking it's the area of your genitalia that you can see if you were inclined to peer at yourself with a mirror. It includes the mons pubis, the labia majora and labia minora (outer and inner 'lips') and the clitoris.

Mons pubis is the fatty padded area of skin that lies over your pubic bone, where all your pubic hair grows. You can find it (if you're really at a loss) about 10cm (4in) below your belly button.

Do use this area to your advantage during sex (see Chapter 3).

Don't shave off all your pubic hair unless you like having itchy stubble down below.

Labia majora are the vaginal lips – the two folds of skin that overlap your vaginal opening.

Labia minora are the small folds of skin found inside the labia majora. In some women they hang down, or protrude from the labia majora, and in others remain hidden in the outer folds.

Do have a look at how this area looks (if you can bear it).

Don't panic if yours don't resemble a textbook drawing of the labia. This whole area greatly varies in shape, size and colour from woman to woman.

Also if you notice a whitish substance, it's worth noting this is just a natural secretion from the sebaceous glands, very similar to smegma which is found under the male foreskin (see page 15) and is easily washed away

Clitoris

The clitoris is actually part of a much bigger organ – we're talking about four inches in length that extends inside you and links to erectile tissue around the vagina. This small organ is the female equivalent of a man's penis, which basically means it comes with its own tiny shaft and glans and it's even covered by a similar piece of skin to the foreskin, known as the hood. The sole purpose of this organ is to give you sexual pleasure.

To locate it, go to the opening of your vagina, where the two inner lips of the labia minora meet. It's worth noting this whole area is also made of similar tissue to the penis, which is why it becomes erect on stimulation and why it feels good when rubbed. When flaccid the average clitoris is the size of a pine nut, and when aroused it swells to the size of a large peanut.

Do feel this area, so you can get used to how you like to be touched here.

Don't panic about the size of your clitoris. It doesn't matter how big or small it is – you can still have an orgasm.

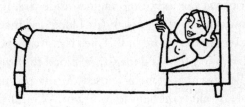

Vagina

The vagina is literally the inside part of your genitalia, the soft muscle-bound canal measuring about three to four inches that has a variety of purposes. Firstly, it's made for penetration by a penis; secondly, it serves as a birth canal for a baby and thirdly, it's the outlet for menstrual blood. At rest the spongy, muscle-bound walls lie flat against each other, but at play the walls stretch and then spring back together afterwards.

Sensitivity-wise the vagina varies greatly; most of the best feelings are to be found on the outer area of the vagina, which is why penile entry can feel so good. The middle area and the area closest to the cervix have much fewer nerves and so you cannot feel much here.

Do expect a normal discharge here at different times of the month.

Don't just shove anything into yourself for 'fun'. A good rule of thumb is if you wouldn't put it in your mouth don't put it in your vagina.

Cervix

Also known as the neck of the womb (uterus), the cervix is located right at the top of the vagina inside you. It's a small, narrow area that is about 2.5cm (1in) long and made of very tough tissue. In the centre of this area is a small opening that allows sperm to get in and menstrual blood to flow out. This is also the area that remains closed during pregnancy and then dilates to allow the baby to come out. All in all, the cervix, though made of strong muscle and tissue, is basically a weak area of the body in terms of cellular activity. This is because during sex two types of cells meet here (yours and his) and this can cause the cells of the cervix to change, which can lead to cervical cancer. One reason why it's essential to go for regular smear tests (see Chapter 7).

Do expect the cervix to be sensitive in a painful way to some deep sexual positions.

Don't stop having sex if you hit the cervix, just change positions.

Uterus

This is your womb – the upside-down pear you learnt about in biology all those years ago. This is the part of your body where a developing foetus lives during pregnancy. The uterus is about 7.5cm (3in) long and 7.5cm (3in) wide and has incredibly powerful muscles – think period pain and the contractions to give birth. During your menstrual cycle this is the area where the endometrium (the lining) builds up and then releases into a period if you're not pregnant.

Do expect some period pain, as the muscles of the uterus are super powerful.

Don't expect period pain to be so bad you can't stand. If it is, see your GP.

Hymen

The thin membrane of tissue that partly covers the entrance to the vagina is called the hymen. This is the ridiculous piece of skin that causes an almighty fuss in some countries as it's supposed to symbolise virginity. The fact is, it's just a membrane and is often torn during strenuous activity or by the insertion of tampons – well before you might have sex.

Do expect to feel a little pain if it breaks the first time you have sex.

Don't expect to notice if it breaks during sport.

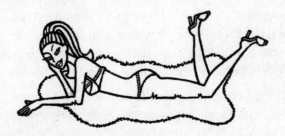

Five supercharged female hot spots

Get him to fondle, stroke, kiss and lick these in the right way and you probably won't need the rest of the book.

1. Breasts

How's his breast action? If it entails a few clumsy gropes and a lot of nipple yanking it's time to take action. Start by getting him to concentrate on the area surrounding your breasts. The area underneath each breast is extra sensitive as is the area of skin to the sides of each boob. Get him to start there and work his way 'slowly' in.

2. The nipple

When he gets to the nipple don't let him do that twiddling thing, instead make him opt for some sucking, kissing and gentle rubbing, making sure he includes the areola (pigmented area of the nipple).

3. Your G-spot

The mysterious G-spot needn't be so mysterious if you let him know what he's looking for. To find it, get him to insert a finger into the vagina and then move upwards 5cm (2in). He should feel the front of the vaginal wall and search for a small textured bump. If he caresses this when you're semi aroused you might be lucky enough to have what's known as a G-spot orgasm – a super-induced orgasm.

facts

Cigarette packs are soon to include warnings that smoking can affect sexual performance, following a European Union decision to put strict new guidelines on packets. This is because smoking causes decreased blood flow to the genital region.

4. Clitoris

This is the female sexual bit that contains the highest concentration of nerve endings in the body. Get him to stimulate this the right way and it's wa-hey! Tips to give him include not touching the area until you are well lubricated, treating it well and applying the right amount of pressure.

5. Perineum

The super-erotic, orgasm-friendly zone found between your vagina and your bottom is the perineum. It's a small patch of lightly ridged skin, small in width, which when rubbed, licked or fondled hits all your pleasure-sensitive nerves in one mighty swoop. If he can't find it with his hand, suggest he goes down and takes a closer look.

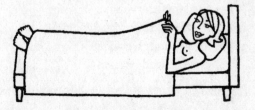

His anatomy bits

Penis

Well, you undoubtedly know what this looks like and you probably also know it's the most sexually sensitive part of the male anatomy. Made up of spongy erectile tissue, involuntary muscle, nerves and blood vessels the penis is more than a simple shaft-shaped organ that hangs partly outside the body, in fact the most interesting stuff goes on inside.

Things You Need to Know:

- The head of the penis (or glans) is highly sensitive. The external urethral opening, through which semen and urine is ejaculated, is at the centre of the glans.
- The average penis is 9cm (3½in) long when flaccid.
- A penis of any size is able to become erect and reach orgasm.
- Size is irrelevant. The truth is, while soft penises look very different, when erect all penises average somewhere between 13 and 18cm (5 and 7in) long.

Penis facts A study by a US condom company, Lifestyles, found that size varies from country to country. In the US the average length is 14.9cm (6in), in Germany 13.9cm (6in) and in Australia and the UK, 12.9cm (5in).

Urethra

This runs from the bladder to the end of the penis.

Things You Need to Know:

- The urethra carries both semen (the fluid that contains sperm) and urine.
- It cannot carry semen and urine at the same time.

Urethra facts During sex, a muscle in the bladder will clamp shut, preventing a flow of urine on ejaculation (the release of semen from the penis).

Foreskin

This is the skin that covers the penis and is folded over the glans and is also known as the head of the penis.

Things You Need to Know:

- Some men have this skin removed for religious or health reasons during childhood.When this happens it's known as circumcision and means the head of the penis is now permanently exposed.
- Circumcision doesn't affect his sexual excitement or yours.
- Uncircumcised men need to be more scrupulous about their personal hygiene to prevent infections of the non-sexual kind. If an uncircumcised man showers regularly, and washes under the foreskin, he'll be as clean and as healthy the next guy.

Foreskin facts The idea that being circumcised is cleaner for women during sex is a myth. A study on circumcision from the University of Chicago found there were no significant sexual-health differences between circumcised and uncircumcised men. The idea that circumcision also prevents cervical cancer has also been disproved by the American Cancer Society.

Testicles

These are two small glands found below the penis.

Things You Need to Know:

- The testicles produce millions of sperm every day.
- They are each about 4cm (1.5in) long and 3cm (1.25in) wide.
- Usually the left testicle hangs slightly lower than the right, to prevent them colliding constantly.
- Each testicle is suspended in the scrotum by a cord known as the spermatic cord. In some cases the balls can twist around and get tangled up. This leads to excruciating pain and nausea and needs urgent medical attention.
- The testicles also produce and secrete the male sex hormone testosterone.
- Never kick someone in the balls for a laugh – a hard, direct blow can tear the wall of the testicles.

Testicle facts Testicular cancer is the most common form of cancer in men aged between 20 and 40 years. Eighty per cent of tumours first appear as swellings in the balls, but 95 per cent of cases can be cured if caught early enough.

"The first time I saw a bloke's penis I was sixteen. I thought it was quite ugly and felt pretty glad I was a girl and didn't have to put up with that all day."

Suzanne, 22

Scrotum

This is the pouch of skin that contains the testicles.

Things You Need to Know:

- The scrotum is baggy, enabling the testicles to hang away from the body because sperm needs to be produced at a temperature 5 degrees lower than the body's normal temperature of 98.6 degrees.

Scrotum facts While the scrotum looks like one sac, it's divided into two areas to house each testicle.

Prostate gland

This lies below the bladder and makes up 30 per cent of the fluid contained in semen.

Things You Need to Know:

- The prostate gland is also known as the male G-spot.
- It's about the size of a walnut.

Prostate facts The gland can produce amazing feelings if

it is directly stimulated. Unfortunately, the only way to get to it is to insert a finger into the anus.

Sperm

Those wriggly tadpole things, called sperm or spermatozoa, are in fact male egg cells. The biological purpose of sperm is to transport genetic information from the male body to the female.

Things You Need to Know:

- The average man produces sperm at a rate of about 1,000 every second.
- It takes about ten weeks for sperm to develop inside the testicles.
- Up to 30 billion sperm are produced each month and 50–100 million can be found in one teaspoon of semen (though 40 per cent will be of no use).

Sperm facts Unlike women, who are born with a certain amount of eggs, men aren't born with sperm. Production doesn't begin until puberty.

Semen

The mixture of fluid and sperm that is ejected from the penis during ejaculation is called semen.

Things You Need to Know:

- Semen is made up of 10 per cent sperm, and 90 per cent fluids (60 per cent from the seminal vesicles and 30 per cent from the prostate gland).

- On ejaculation the average amount dispelled is usually about one teaspoonful.

Semen facts Contrary to popular belief, semen is not full of calories. It contains proteins and vitamins, and between 10 and 30 calories per ejaculation.

Five supercharged male hot spots

The fastest way to his heart…

1. Penis

Lots of men are very touchy about the tip of the penis because it's incredibly sensitive and all men fear pain. So be extra careful, never leap on the penis with teeth bared or apply too much pressure with your tongue. As for a good oral job, keep your teeth covered, don't suck too hard and never bite or grab on too hard (see Chapter 3 for more).

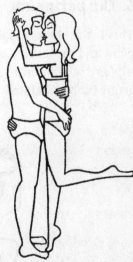

2. Male nipples

Though highly sensitive, not all men like the idea of being touched here. If you do go near, go slowly, never twiddle them and use your tongue. Watch his reaction; if he grimaces, move on.

3. The frenulum

This is a small, ridged area of skin on the underside of the penis. It's an essential spot to go for during sex, as it's an arousal hot spot.

4. The male G-spot

Also known as the prostate gland, to get there you have to stick your finger up his bum (which not all guys like, so always ask first).

5. The perineum

This is the erotic, orgasm-friendly zone found between the penis and the anus, a sort of small patch of skin. It's richly supplied with pleasure-sensitive nerves, and men like it to be gently rubbed and stroked.

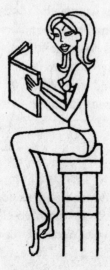

What drives us to have sex?

Sex is a funny thing when you think about it. Two naked bodies humping and sweating their way to supposed bliss. If we didn't all do it the chances are we'd condemn it as pretty base and vulgar. The thing that stops us from turning our noses up are the factors that drive us to have sex. The primary ones of which are our sex hormones. These are the sneaky chemical messengers, which go off like fireworks in our brain, prompting everything from our sexual feelings to emotions and moods. Learn to know how they work, and you can use them to your advantage.

The sexed-up mighty male hormone — testosterone

Testosterone is the sexually predatory hormone, which rules all men. For starters guys carry around 20–40 times as much of it as us females, which is bad news for them, as testosterone is extremely sensitive to its environment. This means waft a DD cup in his face, stick him in a male-only sports environment and/or watch him interact with a group of women and his testosterone will whip around madly, changing his moods and his behaviour on the spot.

Under normal everyday conditions, it's worth noting that testosterone is higher in the morning (as you can probably tell), lower in the late afternoon (when he starts to get tired) and very low at night (when he needs to sleep). It then fluctuates up and down in-between.

6 ways to deal with his hormones

1. Don't Pick on Him
When he's down his testosterone levels will plummet leaving you with a surly, depressed human doormat with no sex drive.

2. Choose Your Time Carefully
Don't demand sexual favours at night when he's tired – it will backfire on you. Go for it in the morning when his sex drive is high.

3. Let Him Help Himself
Don't be put off if he masturbates as well as having sex with you. Kick-starting testosterone surges not only increases the sex drive but also increases the desire to masturbate.

4. Get Him Moving
Taking regular exercise not only promotes the production of all the body's sex hormones, but it boosts testosterone's efficiency.

5. Show Him You're Hot for Him
If he's feeling sexually sluggish show him you're weak with lust and desire for him. This will make his testosterone link up with two other hormones known as LHRH and DHEA (both of which will help boost his flagging sex drive) and translate desire into hot action.

6. Have More Sex

Sex encourages the brain to stimulate production of testosterone, not only in the testicles but also in the brain. Therefore, the more sex you have, the more sex he'll want.

The female hormones — oestrogen and progesterone

If you think the male sex hormone is bad news, take a look at the female ones — oestrogen and progesterone. Oestrogen is the sultry sex kitten of hormones, sexy, vivacious and desperate for attention. While progesterone is the soggy wet blanket, eager to smother those flames of passion and spoil all your fun. These are just two of the shifting hormones which influence our sexual moods every day of the menstrual month. Work out what time of the month you're at and you'll understand the rise and fall of your sex drive.

Days 1—7

Expect to Feel:

Like you've just awoken from a nightmare. Unlike the previous seven days, you should be feeling relaxed, happy and calm. This is all down to the release of a hormone from the brain's pituitary gland called FSH (follicle-stimulating hormone). This hormone stimulates your ovaries and leads to the production of the female sex hormone — oestrogen.

This is a Good Time to:
- Start socialising.

This is Not a Good Time to:
- Go on a manhunt.
- Indulge in a mega sex session.

Days 7–14

Expect to Feel:
Sexy. If days 1–7 have you being the calm in the eye of the storm, days 7–14 will cast you into the storm. This is the highlight of your sexual month, which means it's time to flex those sexual muscles. Thanks to oestrogen you'll be at your most attractive right now. On the sexual front, this means you'll pursue anyone you fancy, enthusiastically and with sex firmly on your mind. However, though your confidence levels will be high, you're low on common sense, so be careful. This is the time you'll catch a real loser and, worse still, it will be another week until you realise it.

This is a Good Time to:
- Have sex.
- Flirt heavily.

Days 14–21

Expect to Feel:
Dull and tired. Days 14–21 are storm-damage days. Initially the LH (lutenising hormone) from the brain will trigger ovulation and boost your libido to an all-time high. However, once ovulation has occurred (one to two days) your oestrogen levels will drop and progesterone will start to rise.

As progesterone is the Mary Whitehouse of hormones, it will kill your rampant sex drive in one fell swoop. On the physical front, you might begin to notice some weight gain, especially around your breasts and stomach (the body begins to store water so you don't get dehydrated before your period arrives). You're also likely to feel flabby and slack off on the exercise front, because progesterone has a sedative effect and your energy levels will be low.

This is a Good Time to:
- Stay at home.
- Have intimate conversations of the 'love' kind.
- Go to bed early.

This is Not a Good Time to:
- Have a series of one-night stands.

facts

There may be a hormonal reason why women need to 'talk' and men need to 'walk' during sexual upsets. Studies from Penn State University, USA, say,'The hormone oxytocin might be the key', as this hormone goes into hyper mode in females during stressful times making us want to talk. Sadly in men it has the opposite effect, enhancing the fight or flight response, urging them to withdraw, get angry or walk away.

Days 21—28

Expect to Feel:
Low. Prepare yourself, because your two favourite sex hormones, oestrogen and progesterone, have dropped out of sight, which means you're likely to feel snappy, irritable, tearful and somewhat depressed.

Not only is this the time when you're likely to buy and wear something you'll live to regret (think canary-yellow cowboy boots), but this is also the time you're most likely to feel blue. This is because your concentration levels are at an all-time low as your body's energies have been processed into other areas of your body. The good news is, with progesterone dropping out of your cycle, testosterone (the male sex hormone) gets a small look-in and, mixed with decreasing levels of oestrogen, this will suddenly give you a sexual surge, which means you'll be incredibly orgasm-friendly!

This is a Good Time to:
- Stay in bed.
- Have an earth-shattering orgasm.
- Eat chocolate.

"My boyfriend says what with my period, PMS and then post-period blues I have about one day a month when I'm in a good mood!"

Tina, 20

What stops you enjoying sex? The sexual demons

Our hormones may drive us to have sex and feel sexy, but sometimes they can be halted by psychological beliefs we hold about sex. So if you feel you're not getting enough out of sex or you feel inhibited about your sexual desires – it's worth bearing in mind the following sexual demons.

Myth: *Sex is dirty*
Only if you want it to be. Joking aside, your upbringing can sometimes hinder your enjoyment of sex and put you off reaching your full sexual potential. Maybe you grew up in a family that believed sex outside of marriage was 'bad' or 'wrong'. Or sex for fun's sake was against a religious belief. If this feels true for you it may be worth considering the fact that sex – as long as it's between two consenting adults – is as natural and as normal as breathing.

Myth: *Women have lower libidos than men*
Well, that's what some men would have us believe. The fact is men and women have the same libidos, it's simply that men are brought up to believe they have a right to have sex, and women aren't. Translated this means some women feel guilty about their desire for sex and so hide it or squash it and forget they have a libido.

Myth: *Men can't be faithful*
Some men can't be faithful and neither can some women – this has little to do with 'biology' and the so-called 'need to

spread their seed' and more to do with their psychological make up.

Myth: *You can't learn to be good at sex*
You can learn to be good at just about everything, especially sex. In fact to be a good lover all you have to do is take the time to learn the moves. After all the best lovers in the world weren't born that way, they were just lucky enough to hook up with someone who could show them the ropes.

Myth: *You should only have sex with someone you love*
Good advice if you can find someone, though it's worth pointing out – good love doesn't equal good sex, and good sex doesn't equal good loving. While a mind–body connection during sex can be amazing, sex for sex's sake is not only more common than you think, but also for many people it is an enjoyable way to pass the time.

Myth: *Only thin people can have good sex*
Good sex isn't dependent on the size of breasts, thighs or stomach (or penis and biceps for that matter). Body size only hinders sex if you are overly self-conscious and try to suck in your stomach halfway through sex or insist on having sex in the pitch dark.

Myth: *You're not a highly sexed person*
Is this true or something you've come to believe because of your current (or past) sex life? The fact is if you're having bad sex you're not going to be highly sexed, in fact, you're probably not going to want to have sex at all. Which is even more reason to experiment and see what's lurking beneath the surface.

Myth: *Sex gets boring in the end for everyone*
Sex only gets boring if you get boring. Meaning if you stop experimenting, trying new things, working on turning each other on and basically trying in and out of bed, your sex life will become dull pretty fast. The good news is sex can be brilliant for the rest of your days as long as you put the effort in.

Why sex is good for us

While I'd be the first to say sex is not the most important thing in life, it's worth considering that having sex does make life more fun. It also happens to be good for your body and health and it beats the heck out of going to the gym every day. Here's what a good bout of sex can do for you.

1. Keep heart disease at bay
A recent study of 2,500 people at the University of Bristol, UK, found that those who had sex at least three times a week lowered their risk of coronary heart disease by 50 per cent. So forget the gym!

2. Increase your longevity
Research at the University of Wales, UK, found people who have two or more orgasms a week tend to live significantly longer than those who avoid both sex and masturbation.

3. Boost your bone strength
Researchers at the University of Virginia, USA, have discovered that regular sex and regular genital stimulation raises levels of the hormone oestrogen in the body. This will help ease PMS symptoms and enhance your mood significantly.

4. Keep you young and beautiful

A study of 3,500 people by scientists at the Royal Edinburgh Hospital, UK, found that those who looked the youngest had the most vigorous sex life.

5. Keep you feeling sexy

Both men and women who have sex often when they are young retain the physical capacity to do so when they are older. Think how quickly your leg would wither if you didn't use it for a few months, well the same applies to your sex drive. If you don't give it regular exercise the capacity for sex when you are older will rapidly fade.

6. Make diets unnecessary

Having regular sex also helps raise levels of the sex hormone DHEA and oestrogen. This in turn lowers cholesterol and causes weight loss without dieting. This is because DHEA and oestrogen affect fat metabolism by triggering what's known as a 'fatty acid cycle', this raises the body's metabolic rate causing you to burn more energy (calories).

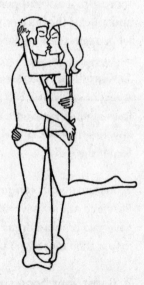

7. Lower your risk of a stroke

Regular sex also results in an overall lowering of blood pressure, which in turn is excellent news for your long-term health. Low blood pressure not only makes your heart beat more efficiently, but it will also help you avoid an age-related stroke.

facts

Starting a new relationship could be the key to a new
sexy body, according to a survey by the UK Health Education Monitoring Survey. It seems people who have
just fallen in love are twice as likely to improve their
diet and gain healthy habits than those who were single
or in a long-term relationship.

8. Help you sleep

Orgasm promotes sounder sleep simply because levels of
the hormone oxytocin peak to five times higher than normal
during orgasm. Sound sleep in turn activates the brain's
neurotransmitters to release the hormone melatonin that
in itself is said to enhance sex and influence depression.
Most importantly of all, melatonin serves as a free-radical
antioxidant (free radicals have been shown to contribute
towards ageing and age-related disease such as osteoarthritis
and cardiovascular disease).

CHAPTER TWO

The solo stuff

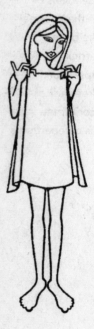

MASTURBATION, SOLO SEX, playing with yourself – call it what you may – these words can make even the strong-hearted sex siren feel faint and giggly simply because when it comes to female masturbation there is still a stigma attached to it. Doing it on your own? Well then, you must be a sad singleton who no one wants to bed, or a nymphomaniac who just can't get enough.

Sound familiar? Well here's the truth – most people, even the laziest lovers, masturbate. This is because for many women, and let's face it for men too, getting off on their own is a pleasure that meets no other. Whatever your preference (and let's face it – some people just don't fancy the idea), having a vibrant solo sex life, whether it's in your head or something more physical, is the key to good sex. Whereas sitting around and waiting for an expert lover to open all your sexual doors is pretty much the sexual kiss of death.

So here's the good news – masturbation, sexual fantasies and having an imaginative and fertile solo sexual life won't ruin you for sex, in fact the opposite has been proven to be true. It also won't make you blind and certainly won't ruin your chances of a future orgasm.

As for how people do it – well, some people go the whole hog, get naked and use the whole of their bodies to get turned on and blissed out. Others don't actually like to touch themselves but masturbate quite effectively through fantasy and genital pressure. Some prefer sex toys (see Chapter 6), and others like quick ones on their own in the office stationery cupboard (if this is you, beware of CCTV cameras).

Whatever your preference, this chapter's for you, because if you want a successful sex life, you need to have a vibrant solo sex life too. Learn what makes your mind and body tick, hum and purr, and I'll guarantee you your lovers will always be back begging for more.

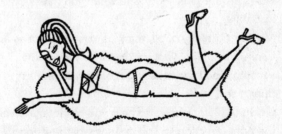

Take a pleasure trip around your body

So why masturbate? Well, top sex experts say, when it comes to sustaining your desire to have sex for life, masturbating regularly is your best insurance policy. This is because masturbation has a variety of benefits for your sex life.

Flying solo gives you...

- A perfect sexual outlet whether you're single or not.
- If you think of your libido as like a muscle, the more you work it the stronger it becomes. Flex your capacity to feel and be sexual and your literal 'love muscles' will keep getting stronger and stronger.
- Sexual benefits aside, masturbation has a variety of health benefits. It not only helps to relieve stress and anxiety but it can also help soothe period pain and kick-start the sleep hormone when you have insomnia.
- Most importantly of all, think of masturbation as a bank investment. What you put into your sexual account, you'll eventually get back with interest during sex.
- Going at it alone will also help you point your lover in the right direction so you can say what feels good, and show him how he can improve his stroke.

If you're still interested here's how to give it a try.

Rule one: *Ignore your rules*
Masturbation is a preference and how you choose to do it is up to you. However, for those stuck at where to go next and feeling faintly ridiculous, all you need to do is basically get your hands moving over your body.

Rule two: *Get private*
Of course it helps if you get private first. So lock the door, because you're not going to feel very sexy if you're afraid someone is going to come barging through at any moment. Also make sure you choose a time and place where you won't be disturbed by noisy flatmates. Turn off your mobile and your answerphone (or you will kill the mood instantly when your mum calls up to leave you a message). Now do what you need to do to feel comfortable. For some people this means turning off the light, for others it means getting naked.

"I can't bear the thought of touching myself. I tried it once and I felt really pervy and stupid. I'm not uptight about sex it's just that masturbating is not for me."

Jacq, 20

Rule three: *Don't just lie there*
Now let your hands wander around, let them graze over various areas. Remind yourself of the hot spots from Chapter 1, and at the same time focus on some of the other

erogenous zones such as your lips, your face and your neck. You may already know the bits that make you tingle and shiver, but getting to grips with some of the not so obvious areas will not only improve how you feel about your body, but also help you boost your hot-lover potential. Above all, remember, this is not a science experiment, so don't treat your body like a slab of meat.

Rule four: *Think sexy thoughts*

If this is the first time you've given this a try, or the first time you've given masturbation a thought, it might help to get in the right mood. For some women this means a sexy movie or an erotic book. If that's not your scene, try to think sexy thoughts as you move around your body, it will help you to feel sexy. Remember past encounters, good ex-lovers (or present ones) or even what turns you on from films you've seen.

The aim here is to let your mind just go for it. Don't feel self-conscious or think about how ridiculous you might look, as this will make orgasm pretty unlikely. Ask yourself:

- Does it feel better when you apply hard pressure or light pressure to your breasts?
- Do you like the feel of your inner thigh being stroked or lightly pinched?
- Does it work for you when you can feel your nipple being rubbed, or stroked?

When you feel ready move this emphasis to your genital region. The following are just some of the ways that women make masturbation work for them.

- Rubbing the clitoris directly with the palm of the hand, or with the fingers.
- Applying pressure to the clitoris with an object such as a pillow or towel.
- Rubbing the clitoris against the mattress.
- Using a vibrator on the clitoris.
- Using a showerhead against the clitoris.
- Penetrating the vagina with fingers.
- Stroking and rubbing the breast, nipple and bottom.
- Playing with the erogenous zones of the body and genitals.

facts

What can relieve a headache, stave off depression, and combat the aches and pains of everyday life? Well, according to a study from the American Association of Sex Educators, the answer is 'genital stimulation'.

Rule five: *Making it work for you*
Tried all of the above and nothing happened? Well don't write it off. Maybe you were expecting too much, or were too tense this time around or something disturbed you. The fact is sometimes masturbation can bring you to orgasm, other times it will just have you hovering on the edge and now and again it won't do anything at all. If this happens, try some problem solving.

- Do you need extra help with some lubrication? This may turn you off, but nothing will spoil your enjoyment faster than rubbing away when it's as dry as a desert down there. So buy some KY jelly.

- Next think about positions. Were you sitting up, lying down, standing up, in a chair? The best position for beginners is usually lying down on your back, with legs apart. If that doesn't work for you and you feel too exposed, try lying on your front, with your head on a pillow. It won't give you easy access to your breasts but will help you to lose yourself in the moment.

- Then try to change the way you touch yourself. Feeling squeamish about penetration? Then don't do it. Hate the pulling sensation when you rub? Then try stroking or circling. Try sliding your fingers down either side or imagine how you'd like someone else to touch you during sex, and do it that way.

- Don't be orgasm obsessed. Studies show most women take about four minutes to come during masturbation, but many women take longer.

- Vary your rhythm. Just as you wouldn't want a lover to grab at your breasts and pound away furiously down below, give yourself a good ride by building up pace and rhythm. Vary your touch speed, and experiment with tension by either keeping your legs straight, or pressing the soles of your feet together.

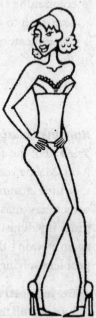

Rule six: *Take it out of the bedroom*
While you'll probably formulate all your best ideas in bed, when you feel confident

it pays to take masturbation off the mattress. While I'm not advocating you go for it in public on the number 37 bus, it can pay to be brave about your solo pursuits. Try it in the bathroom, in the shower, sitting in a chair opposite a long mirror, standing up, with clothes on, and even with your lover during sex. The latter may sound scary but mutual masturbation will not only enhance your sex life but it can also prolong sex and help you to achieve orgasm every time you have sex.

facts

New research shows if you want better moves and orgasms in bed, the best person to practise on is yourself. The research from the John Hopkins University, USA, points out that if you experiment with varying ways of coming when you're alone you are more likely to become an expert at sex, and get exactly what you want in bed.

Male masturbation

A few words about what he gets up to on his own.

It may sound sexist but as men have less of a stigma attached to their solo pursuits they're usually pretty skilled in handling themselves by the time they reach 14, never mind 25 years old. This means by the time you get hooked up with a guy, the chances are he'll be an expert in his field. On the whole for most men, masturbation happens pretty fast, pretty much daily and has little bearing on whether they are attached, single or having sex with someone. This means they know exactly how to direct you to what works and what doesn't (another reason to take a leaf out of their book).

Solo flights can teach men...

- How to prolong orgasm.
- How the point of no return feels (important for your sex life).
- What makes them come faster and what turns them on.
- It's also a way of relieving boredom, taking away sexual frustration and generally de-stressing.

How men do it

Men usually start by thinking of something that turns them on, and as guys are more open and honest than us about being visually stimulated, they use a variety of 'tools', maybe a sexy video or a porn magazine, though many just use their minds. On the whole, male orgasm comes from stimulating the penis, so common ways a guy may masturbate include:

- Using a fast rubbing movement on the shaft of their penis with their hand.
- Focusing on the head (glans) of the penis – an area crammed full of nerve endings. He might just apply pressure here or alternate between a back and forth movement on the shaft and then some head action.

- A vigorous stroking action all over and a rubbing on the scrotum and testicles.
- Stimulation of the perineum and his thighs and bottom.
- Pulling back the foreskin and building up a rhythm and fast pace.
- Some men also use lubrication to help them build up friction.

The whole process only takes a few minutes, which is also why some men have a problem with premature ejaculation – see Chapters 3 and 7.

Troubleshooting

Now you've got to grips with masturbation it pays to be aware of the following because while solo ventures are great for you and your sex life, they won't be if you take it all too seriously.

- Vary what you do when you're on your own. If you teach your body to orgasm only when you go through a certain routine, your body will start to react only to that pattern. This can spell trouble in the bedroom. Remember masturbation is the key to good sex, not the only way to good sex.
- Don't fake it and then secretly make it on your own. While it's great that you can have a good solo journey it doesn't pay to make yourself feel better after bad sex by masturbating. Don't wait for him to roll over and start snoring, if sex hasn't done it for you, take his hand and show him what needs to be done.
- Don't be freaked out by the intensity of his solo orgasm. Most men tend to grip themselves quite tightly when they

are masturbating. This equals a strong orgasm, something that can't be replicated by the vagina.

- Don't be freaked out by his technique. Remember, masturbation is a guide to improving sex, not a road map with markers on.

- Given it a try and still hate it? Then stop – you don't have to go solo, in fact you don't have to do anything you feel uncomfortable with when it comes to sex. Instead see below and concentrate on the mind–body fantasy element in your solo sex life.

- Don't imagine his solo pursuits will stop when he starts having sex with you. He's been doing it for years and is likely to see no problem in carrying on while you're together. It's not a sign you're not enough for him in bed, and you shouldn't view it as a problem unless he's opting for masturbation over sex. After all, what's stopping you from carrying on too? Masturbation, as we've said before, will improve your sex life, boost your libido and keep you feeling sexual.

> "I remember one ex walking in on me going for it and freaking out. It was as if she thought masturbation was the same as having an affair and wouldn't speak to me for days. How weird is that?"
>
> **Tom, 25**

Do it together

The trick is to bring what you've learnt about yourself into your sex life because unless you're dating a mind reader the chances are your boyfriend's never going to work out what's going on in your sexual head. The sexiest and laziest way for both of you to discover what makes the other tick is to try masturbating together. Apart from the fact that sex talk is a hundred times easier when you're both naked and in the mood, mutual masturbation is less embarrassing than you might imagine. The chances are you probably do it already or have done it. (Remember your pre-sex encounters? Well, that's what we're talking about.) Here are a variety of ways to try it out – choose the one that makes you feel the least self-conscious.

Watching each other

Benefits: An excellent way of seeing how your partner likes to be touched and played with; high arousal potential. On the whole men are more confident about showing you their bits before you show them yours. It sounds silly especially if you already have an active sex life, but being brave enough to show him all your solo secrets can be tough. If you're feeling shy about it, let him go first. When it's your turn return the favour, imagine you're putting on a show for him. Keep semi-dressed if that makes you feel better and tell him what you're doing and why. Not only will it be a huge turn-on for him, but a very good lesson in how he can improve his foreplay style. Help yourself by:

- Paying attention to what he does and the pace and rhythm he builds up as he reaches orgasm.
- Showing him what you're happy with and what area of his technique you're not so keen on.
- Making some noise. You may know exactly what all that rubbing's doing for you, but he may not be able to read your signals. Moan, sigh and whimper louder so he gets your message.
- Watching carefully. Unsure of how to give him a good hand job? This will show you without you having to ask.
- Not being orgasm obsessed. Is he penis-fixated or is he moving further afield?
- Not just focusing on your own genitals. Show him your other hot spots – your breasts, your neck, anywhere that you also like to be stroked.
- Refusing to be self-conscious. Get him involved, put his hands over yours, tell him what you're thinking, allow him to take over.
- Making this sexual play a part of your normal sex life.

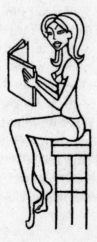

facts

Any form of genital contact, whether or not it results in an orgasm, is an ideal way of releasing endorphins (the body's natural painkillers) and blocking off pain.

Mutual masturbation

Benefits: A more physically intense orgasm brought about simply by touch; a bigger chance of a simultaneous orgasm especially if he starts on you first.

Mutual masturbation is when you both touch each other at the same time. This allows both of you to get your juices going super fast and to achieve orgasm. The aim is to do it all through touch. So use your hands, lips, mouth and voice, and explore each other's bodies. Remember to concentrate on all the erogenous areas you've already located on your own body, plus some of the following:

1. The side panels
These are two highly irresistible and frequently overlooked zones literally on the sides of your body. You can find the exact spot, by skimming 5cm (2in) just below your armpit and stroking up and down. When touched here, expect to feel your stomach do a little flip and tingly sensations run up and down your spine. This area's hot, because it's crammed full of nerve endings and rarely touched. To get the feeling, get him to caress the area gently with long, lightly pressured strokes. If he's too rough you'll lose the sensation. If he does it right you'll be writhing with joy all over the bed.

2. Earlobes

Extra, extra-sensory spots. This spot is so highly sex-charged that rubbing, nibbling and stroking here will send frantic, 'Yes! Yes!' messages to your brain. But be warned, when you're using this in sex, contrary to popular myth, an ear saliva bath does not feel sexy.

3. Fingers and hands

The fingers are highly sensitive because they have a fast track directly to the brain. Try tender stroking, or a mouth-sucking moment. For maximum effect, suggest he tries drawing one or two fingers into his mouth slowly and sucking suggestively. Apart from giving you an idea of his general technique down below, it will also give you direct eye-to-eye contact with him while he does it – too sexy for words!

4. Feet and lower legs

The soles of the feet and the spaces between the toes have a super strong connection to your sex organs. Rubbing here will stimulate your sex organs faster than a quick grope. To send those sexual currents straight to the right place, get him to gently push a finger between two toes and move it around slowly. You'll immediately feel sexually squishy because this tender, soft bit craves attention and fondling. Lastly make sure he encircles your ankles with small kisses and strokes up your calves towards your knees – another sizzling spot.

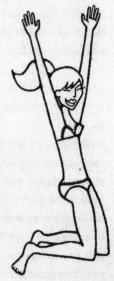

5. Inner thigh

It's likely you already know about this one, but did you know you can actually reach the big O by simple hand-to-thigh stimulation and nothing else? Again this has a lot to do with nerve endings, but also much to do with sexual anticipation. What could be better than feeling hot breath and inquisitive fingers play up and down your inner thigh. Get him to tease you with long, massaging strokes, and if you can bear it, a light tickling caress. No cheating though!

6. Hair

Ever wondered why you like running your own fingers through your hair? Well, it's because gently pulling hair massages the scalp and energises the body. If you want to feel a sexual sensation as well, you need to ensure two things. One, your bloke knows the difference between gently pulling hair and yanking hair. Next, it helps if your hair is tangle free and he can easily run his hands through it. To achieve the full sexual sensation, get him to start at the base of your scalp on the sides of your head and work inwards. Gently running a hand up through your hair and back towards your neck, massaging and kissing your neck on the way down.

7. Spine

Ever had a massage? Well, if you have, you don't need me to tell you the spine is littered with hundreds of tiny erogenous zones, many at the base of the spine. Suggest he drives you wild by moving in small circular movements away from the neck all the way down to your bottom. Then get him to run his hands up and down your spine. Trailing his fingers along your spine as if he were playing a piano. This will not only get your juices flowing, but also cause the nerves in your back to go crazy with desire. For an extra boost get him to lie partially on you while he massages your shoulders and the top of your spine.

8. Behind the knees and wrists

These are frequently ignored sex zones, which is a shame because they are strong pulse points. Roughly translated this means a spot of kissing, stroking and/or sucking will have your blood pooling in exactly the right area, heating the area up, making it throb and having you in a nice rosy glow... need I go on?

9. Your inner forearms

Body-language experts say the forearms are a huge sexual plus area because they are rarely touched and rarely seen. Think about it, how often are the undersides of your arm viewed? So roll up your sleeves and get him to stroke and kiss the soft underbelly of your arm. Expect to feel mega turned on, and for an extra buzz get him to rub his face and lips over the area slowly and tantalisingly.

10. Your tummy

Another frequently missed hot spot, usually because you're too busy sucking it in to let him play with it. However, letting him roam this area with his fingers and lips is pretty darn hot! If you can bear it, let him investigate your belly button (it will send tiny shivers down your body). One word of warning if he's going for a tummy massage make sure he does it in a clockwise direction (or else it will mess up your digestion) and also make sure you are relatively wind free before he starts.

Fantasies – working out what turns you on

Masturbation isn't the only way to get your juices flowing in under a minute. The good old-fashioned fantasy is perhaps your most powerful arousal tool. If you want to be turned on for the rest of your life at the flick of a switch, your aim should be to build up a library of erotic encounters, scenarios and downright sexy stories that you can draw on whenever you are alone or with someone.

In the best-known book on women's fantasies – *My Secret Garden*, by Nancy Friday – women from all over the world talk about what does it for them. Inside you'll find everything from the slave-girl fantasy to fake rape scenarios, to everyday encounters that you'd laugh your head off at if you saw it replicated on TV. And that is the pure pleasure of fantasy – it's not real, it doesn't have to stand up to real life, and you certainly don't have to re-enact it in life.

The whole point is to have your very own sexual turn-on to draw on. A good sexy scenario should put you centre stage (if that's what does it for you) and make you feel sexy pretty instantaneously. While masturbation and fantasies go hand in hand, it's worth noting that drawing on a hot sexual fantasy can help during sex, especially if you're having trouble hovering on the brink of orgasm or are with someone who has the sexual imagination of a slug.

How we form our sex dreams

Sexperts believe fantasies are formed in our head as we grow up and are taken from things we have seen, read about and maybe even gone through. That aside, they could just be things that titillate and excite you for no other reason than they're naughty and a bit taboo. Whatever the reasoning behind your sexual daydreams, if you feel guilt about your fantasies don't obsess about it – all these daydreams represent are mental images that you use to enhance your sex life. They aren't real, don't mean you're a pervert and certainly aren't indications of what you'd really like to do.

What women want in fantasies

- To be taken by a stranger.
- To be with someone famous.
- To have a threesome.
- To have sex with another woman.
- To have someone watch them.
- To be punished/spanked.

Some people have a consistent theme to their fantasies, while others change theirs all the time. Studies, however, show there are certain common patterns and themes that come up in fantasies for both men and women. These tend to be being with someone famous, being forced, being submissive and being dominated or dominating. Take a look at some common male and female themes.

A common unifying fact in all fantasies is that although men tend to play with images that are more visual (think pornographic), both men and women tend to focus on things they'd like to do or try at least in their heads. Still worried about what's going through his head? Here are some myths about fantasies that are worth destroying.

Myth: *I dream about women – I must be gay*
Not at all (unless, of course, you know you are). Same-sex fantasies are a way of playing with an idea and don't mean anything besides the fact you're curious. If, of course, you fancy women, think you're going out with the wrong sex and are desperate for a homosexual experience, then, and only then, will this fantasy mean more.

Myth: *I fantasise about other men during sex so I must leave my boyfriend*
Ask any couple who has been with each other for years and they'll both admit that now and then they'd much rather pretend they were having sex with a film star than their partner. It doesn't mean they want to run off with a movie star, it's just a secret way of spicing up a long-running sex life for the night. It's nothing to feel guilty about unless of course you do it every single time you have sex, and really do want to leave your partner.

Myth: *Odd fantasies mean you're odd*
There's a big difference between dreaming and fantasising about odd and nutty stuff and wanting to do odd and nutty stuff in real life. Some people fantasise about being tied naked to a tree by pirates and being 'saved' by a knight – it's weird but it doesn't mean they're weird. The only time you should worry is if your fantasies scare you or you feel compelled to act out something that could potentially hurt you (in a bad way) or hurt someone else. If this is what you mean by 'odd'

then it's worth going to speak to a trained professional just to put your mind at rest.

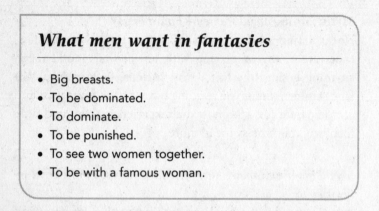

What men want in fantasies

- Big breasts.
- To be dominated.
- To dominate.
- To be punished.
- To see two women together.
- To be with a famous woman.

Myth: *Men always imagine they're with other women*
Also untrue. Ask most men what they're thinking of during sex and the answer is usually sex. For men sex means being very much in the moment – unlike women, their minds aren't really racing around picking out scenarios from their fantasy library but focusing on their orgasm. Even if he is thinking about other women during foreplay, it doesn't mean he's being unfaithful – like most people playing around with images, they can add extra pep to a sexual encounter. It's all part of sex play – and means nothing else at all.

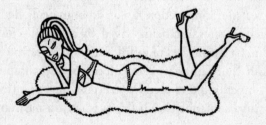

Sexual turn-offs

Finally, just as there are a whole wealth of situations, scenarios and people that will turn you on in life, there are also an equal number of sexual turn-offs. While these will be unique to you – and you are entitled to hold these beliefs and act on them – there are a few turn-offs which can hinder your sex life if you don't act on them.

The anti-sex brigade

Hopefully, being a sex siren, you'll never come across a member of this section of the population. These are the people who think sex is a dirty word – something not to be enjoyed, and certainly not to be had outside of marriage. Maybe you have been brought up with these beliefs. If so, it could be a main factor in why you find sex difficult and uncomfortable. If this is you, it can pay to see someone to talk about the sexual messages you've been taught. A qualified therapist can help talk through your beliefs about sex and help free you from the limiting ones.

Bullying lovers

These are lovers who try to get you to stick to their rules. It usually occurs when you meet someone who assumes he is more experienced than you are and so wants you to do things his way. When it comes to sex, the rule is simple – only do things you want to do. As we said earlier – masturbation isn't for everyone, neither are some sexual moves, certain fantasies and certain types of sexual behaviour. Lack of experience has little to do with what you feel is a turn-on and what is a turn-off. Be true to yourself with sex, otherwise you'll turn yourself off for good.

Being wild when you're not

Like the above, a pressure to perform can be the ultimate turn off when it comes to sex. Magazines, and even books can all add to the feeling that somehow if you're not wild and experimental you're a sexual dud in bed. Luckily this is not so. Studies show most people don't bother with Olympic-style sexual positions, but stick to the good old missionary one. Plus most of us aren't having sex in scary public places, but do it in the bedroom, and the sauciest most women get is to buy raunchy underwear from M&S! This is not because we're all boring and dull (because let's face it who knows what you might do with sexy undies on) but because being wild isn't a turn-on for everyone. If you do have a wild streak it's also worth noting that it's always best to bring it out gradually especially if you don't want to frighten a new lover away (see Chapter 6 for more details).

A word about pornography

Does the thought of pornography leave you cold? Or maybe it leaves you feeling hot. The fact is pornography isn't a black-and-white subject. Some women feel it's degrading and only for seedy sad men in raincoats, while others get a thrill from looking at it. Whatever your feelings about porn it's worth noting it's often a guy's first port of call in the sex stakes as a teenager. Meaning you're unlikely to meet many guys who haven't at least taken a look at top-shelf mags and videos. In fact he could still be using it now. So if you're desperate to know, ask him.

"When I was eight my friend and I secretly took a look at a porn mag we found and were totally disgusted by the pics. I remember thinking — 'Yuck — what on earth is going on between the women's legs? I'm never going to go near there in my life.' "

Mark, 20

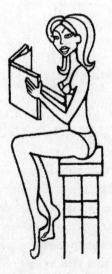

The answer you'll get to this question depends on: (1) the tone of your voice, and (2) whether or not you already know the answer to this question. If you've been snooping and have found a box filled with ten years' worth of his porn magazines, it's likely your aim is to make him feel like a sad loser. If so, it's worth noting the following:

- Most men and lots of women use porn as visual stimuli both together and alone.
- As long as he's not forcing you to look at it, he's not obsessed by it and it's not violent and sick – it's up to him.
- Make him throw it away and he won't thank you or think much of you. In fact he'll probably still use it behind your back.
- Of course, if you're asking because you want to indulge with him, then ask away.

CHAPTER THREE

The sex stuff

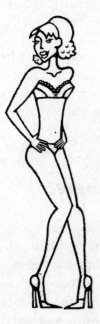

WHAT MAKES FOR GOOD SEX for lazy girls? A multiple orgasm without having to lift a finger? A boyfriend who can't get enough of you or do enough for you? Sex wherever and whenever you want it? All of these things, or none of them? Well, the definition of good sex is different for everyone so whether you're currently getting some or not, it's worth noting that clocking up numbers of bed partners you've had, or the times you've screamed the house down are not ideal indications of whether you've had excellent sex.

If you want to boost your in-bed moments – here's how.

The art of oral sex

The good news about oral sex is if you're on the receiving end there's not much to do but lie back and enjoy! Probably a big component of why people love it so much. Other reasons why people love it are:

- It often feels more intimate than penetration.
- Orgasm is more likely to occur.
- Being felt with someone's tongue is unlike any other sensation you'll feel.
- It feels naughty.
- There's no risk of getting pregnant.
- It's the fastest way to get someone aroused for sex.

However, if you're the giver then there's much work to be done because it's worth noting that though zillions of people are willing to go south in the name of good sex, good oral sex rarely comes easily for anyone. If you're unsure of how to give a blow job successfully here are some pointers.

Do you really want to go there?

This is the first question you should be asking yourself. He may expect you to just do it, but if it's a turn off you need to work out why. Many women don't like giving head (fellatio) because they are worried about doing it wrongly. Others worry about smells, gagging halfway though and whether they should swallow or not. If this is your fear, bear in mind there are no rules to oral sex. Just do what you feel comfortable with.

Is his sexual hygiene up to scratch?

Even the most wanton of lovers will become unresponsive fast when faced with horrible personal hygiene. If you come up from between his legs making gagging noises and holding your nose, the chances are he's not as clean as he could be. Don't feel embarrassed about mentioning this, as hygiene is the number-one reason women avoid oral sex. If you're too scared to say, 'You stink', good tactics include:

- Dragging him into the shower under the guise of foreplay.
- Buying him a spa day at his gym.
- Suggesting a long bath frolic.

Warning

If he still smells ripe despite washing, then it's likely he's going to give you more than an orgasm (i.e. an STI or bacterial infection). If this is the case, your best bet is to slap on a condom asap and make an appointment for both of you at your local genito-urinary medicine clinic (see Chapter 7).

Forget about deep-throating

This is a sad 1970s porn film idea that just doesn't work (unless you're a sword swallower). As we all have a gag reflex at the back of our throats the only reaction he'll get if he tries to go for this is you hurling your guts up.

Worried about the taste

Semen is a mix of sperm, protein, sugars and fluid, and contrary to popular belief is not calorific. It can taste a bit odd: sometimes it's salty, other times it's affected by what your man's eaten. Other than that it's nothing to get hysterical about.

The ultimate guide to giving oral sex

Just thinking about you going down on him can make a man wild with lust for you. Why? Well, because the penis is the male sex organ, which means it's full of nerve endings, so he's guaranteed an orgasm. Plus, men say they like nothing better than to see you giving them direct penile stimulation. If you want to enjoy the encounter as much as him, try the following:

1. Get comfy
There's nothing worse than being in an awkward position for oral sex. So place yourself in the right spot. He can sit or stand, and you can kneel in front of him, or he can lie back on the bed so your head is between his thighs.

2. Don't let him hold your head
This is the biggest complaint from women about blow jobs. You should always control the pace and depth of his penis, so never let him hold your head and do the controlling.

3. Start with your hands
Stroke his penis with your hands so he begins to get aroused. Now before you place your lips around him, make a fist and

place it around the base of his penis. This will stop him thrusting into your mouth and help you to guide his penis where you want it to be. If he thrusts get him to lie on his back so you are more in control.

4. Lick it

Treat him like a lollypop – don't just suck but lick and kiss. Try licking the length from base to head, use the tip of your tongue or the flat part (these will give him different sensations). Curl your tongue round him, and then focus on the head. Special attention should be given to the area of ridged skin under the head, known as the frenulum, as this is extra sensitive. The best move for the head of the penis is to move your mouth up and down and suck gently.

"Some girls are so frightened of oral sex and hand jobs. They just go at it too lightly and it just doesn't work. Firmness is the answer – go for it girls we love it when you do."

Max, 24

5. Add a twist

Spice things up by using a flavoured lubricant or a strong mint. This helps the mouth to water and the minty flavour warms the penis as you place your lips around him.

6. Use your hands

Worried about jaw ache? Then use your hands as well. If your mouth is focusing on the head of his penis, use your hands to work the base and caress and hold his testicles at the same time (though check if he likes this). You could also try rubbing the perineum (the small ridge of skin between the penis and anus), as this will generate more sexual excitement for him.

7. Don't forget the rest of his body
You may be giving him oral but you can still stroke, caress and touch the rest of his body. Focus on his thighs and his bottom and even his anus for extra effect. The aim with oral sex is to make love with your mouth, so for an all-over experience, keep your hands and lips moving all over.

facts

Findings at the World Congress of Sexology found that UK women do not rate sex as important as Europeans. Only 22 per cent of UK women had sex more than once a week compared to 34 per cent of French women.

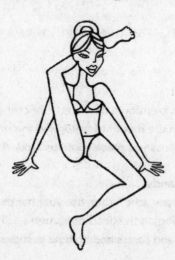

8. To spit or swallow

You don't have to swallow if you don't want to – it doesn't make you a crap lover. Just keep some tissues nearby and spit if he comes in your mouth. Try to do it politely, after all it's not sexy to see your lover coming up and running to the bathroom. If you don't want this to happen, look out for signs that he's going to ejaculate. Just before he does (and he should be able to warn you) his hips should retract a little, his penis will swell and contort, and his balls will move closer to the body. If you can't spot physical signs, then listen to his breathing and note how his thrusting pattern speeds up.

Worries about receiving oral sex from him

Many women would quite happily give oral sex but feel weird about receiving cunnilingus from their boyfriends. Popular worries include:

- Fears your genitals smell.
- Fears he doesn't really want to do it.
- Worries that you won't come.
- Fears you don't know how to respond to sensations.
- Fears you have odd-looking genitalia.

The good news is that none of the above is true. While the vagina does have a natural musty smell, it's not disgusting and should not smell fishy (if it does you probably have a slight infection and need to have it checked out – see Chapter 7). Also bear in mind at certain times of the month, the vagina will have different levels of lubrication – all it takes is good hygiene to ensure that none of these things are a problem. As for the look of your genitalia – don't worry, like the eyes, ears and nose everyone's sex bits look different.

As for cunnilingus, it's worth knowing most women have orgasms more easily from this than any other sex act simply because of the direct stimulation to the clitoris.

Good oral sex on women should include:

- Stimulation of the clitoris, the length of the vagina and the perineum.
- Stimulation of the inner thighs and breasts.
- Focus and attention on the clitoris.
- Use of hands for penetration, and stimulation.
- A steady and even-paced rhythm with his tongue.
- A certain amount of direction from you (if you're too embarrassed to say anything try moaning appreciatively or moving him to the right place by shifting your body).
- A willing lover.

Oral troubleshooting

1. The 69 position doesn't work for you

Lots of people don't like the 69 position for a variety of different reasons. Some people can't get comfortable; others find it hard to orgasm. The most popular complaint from women is they find giving and receiving at the same time distracting and so can't focus on having an orgasm. Men also complain that they don't get the right kind of oral sex because their girlfriends are distracted. The reason being if you're approaching orgasm you're literally not going to be able to focus on the job at hand, and if you are concentrating on the job at hand, you're less likely to have an orgasm. It's a vicious circle, and if this is the case your best bet is to stay in the 69 position but go at it one at a time. This way you can give the way you want, and receive without any distraction whatsoever.

2. You'd rather give a good hand job than mouth job

This is a good alternative to oral sex. Tips for success include:

- Don't grab on too hard and pull – this is the number-one complaint from guys about hand-job techniques. The penis looks strong but it's hypersensitive when erect.
- Ask him to show you what he likes; it beats having to rub the skin raw on your hand. Every bloke is different – some like a strong grip, others a lighter but faster movement. Get them to start, and put your hand over his to get the right feel.
- Once you're on track about the amount of pressure and rhythm he likes, try using both hands and go from the base of the penis all the way to the ridge at the head applying slightly more pressure at the head and at the base for an extra twist.
- Use lubrication as this will help warm up the penile shaft and keep the motion smooth. Try KY jelly or saliva.
- Get into it – doing it looking bored or yawning won't speed up his orgasm or do anything for you in the arousal stakes.
- As soon as he orgasms – let go as the head of the penis can become very sensitive like the clitoris.

3. You hate too much focus on your clitoris during oral sex

This is also fairly common. It occurs because the clitoris sometimes disappears right before orgasm as it retracts and gets lost as the labia swells; men then give too much focus in trying to find it. It also becomes hypersensitive because all the nerve endings are on red alert (some men find this with the head of the penis). If this is the case, just get your lover to back off and be gentle.

4. You don't know what to do with the foreskin

Well, you don't have to do anything. However, pulling the foreskin tight over the shaft can increase the pleasure for men. The best way to do this is to make a ring shape round the end of the penis – about 2.5cm (1in) away from the base – and then pull down so the upper part of the penis is slightly exposed. Or you could try licking round the foreskin and focusing on the head of the penis.

"*Most guys get oral sex so wrong. They just dive down and slobber away as if they're trying to lap up a bowl of milk. It's really off-putting and annoying. It's like they think you should be grateful no matter what they're doing down there.*"

Lola, 24

5. Your boyfriend won't go down on you

There are many reasons why a man says he won't go down on a woman. Reasons such as, 'It's dark and I can't see what I'm doing', 'It feels odd' and the ridiculous, 'It smells.' The truth is most guys who steer clear of oral sex do so because they're scared of doing it wrong and for no other reason.

Which means if you want your guy to go down on you, the best way to do it is to tell him why and exactly how you like it.

This will work immediately because: (1) there's no way he'll be able to misinterpret your request, and (2) your A–Z directions will equal a spot-on delivery. Include as many visual descriptions as you can, as this is how a guy will work out how to do it. Make sure you include the fact that you need a consistent and regular rhythm, a gentle, not rough, pressure and stimulation right through to orgasm.

Having sex Part 1 – foreplay

You don't need me to tell you how to have sex. You just get your clothes off, go for penetration, give it a few thrusts and you're done aren't you?

Hopefully you shouted a resounding 'No' to that one.

The fact is while the act of sex is simple, having good sex isn't. Which is why it's essential to combine everything you now know about sex. Think biology basics, solo pursuits, mental turn-ons, foreplay tips, erogenous zones and oral sex. It's these things that will all lead you towards having better sex and maybe even having an orgasm. If you are too penetration obsessed, you can still have the sex but it won't be as exciting or as long. Want some fast, lazy-girl tips on good foreplay? Look no further.

Good foreplay should contain:

- More than five minutes of pre-penetrative sex.
- Lots of kissing and holding.
- Mutual touching of bodies and exploring.
- Fervent licking and nibbling.
- A general all-over body feel or grope.
- Coverage of most of the erogenous zones (see Chapter 2).
- Oral sex of some kind.
- Some talking (but not too much, as a running commentary is very unsexy).
- Use of hands, fingers, tongues and lips and anything else you can think of.

Improve your foreplay by:

1. Doubling the amount of time you spend on it

If your boyfriend's a sprinter, take control and work on building the pre-penetration stage, by getting him to focus on what he's doing, not where he's going. Most guys rush from start to climax not because they're eager for penetration, but because they're hopeless at foreplay and have no idea what to do once they've given your boobs a few tweaks. Help him by showing him there's more to foreplay than kissing, nipple play and a few body fumbles. Start and prolong the action with some simple kissing.

2. Being sexy about taking your clothes off

While ripping clothes off can be hot, letting him fumble about with your bra for ten minutes, getting your head stuck in your jumper and catching his penis in his flies are big arousal killers. Don't be so eager to get naked, clothes are sexier than you think. Work on the striptease element to really get him going. Get him to watch you slowly peel your clothes off, or better still lie there in your underwear and watch him strip for you.

3. Asking him what he likes

Men are notoriously deficient in the sexual communication department, so if you don't ask, he's likely to use underhand methods to get you where he wants. Do not allow any pushing of the head southwards, or any body flipping, as this will kill the moment. Instead get him to ask/beg/work for what he wants. It will not only up his arousal but increase the sexiness value of what's going on.

4. Not expecting him to be a mind reader

In the same way as above, ask and ye shall receive is the key to getting what you want. Need more oral, less kissing, more licking? Then tell him what you're yearning for from him. At the same time, if words fail you then think about using the whole of your body to turn him on and point him in the right direction. Think fingers, lips and tongue, and try for hands-on penetration, as this can bring you to orgasm.

5. Refusing to fake it

If something's not working for you, say so, otherwise you can expect a lifetime of the same technique. Blokes work on the if-it's-not-broke-don't-fix-it principle, meaning if you don't tell him you hate him licking your ear, he's going to keep doing it until you go bonkers.

6. By not being clueless about foreplay

Finally, remember foreplay counts, but not when it's crap. A cack-handed attempt at oral sex, a slap on the butt and a half-baked attempt at sexual massage is not quality technique. Stuck for ideas? Then read up on what can liven sex up (see Chapters 2 and 6).

Having sex Part II – losing your virginity

Virginity is one of those use and/or abuse terms. Basically despite the hype and myth it's not an indication of the type of person you are, only that you haven't had sex yet. It doesn't mean you'll be a crap lover or that you won't be able to have an orgasm (after all, let's face it, you're probably not a virgin, as in a beginner, in other sexual areas), or even that you'll be better in bed than someone who's been at it for years. As for the idea that everyone is doing it – figures from the Office for National Statistics in the UK show that while around a quarter of all British girls lose their virginity before the age of 16 years, the majority wait until they are around 19 years. So for those currently considering first-time sex, here's all you'll ever need to know about losing it:

1. Accept it might be harder than you think

Lots of first-time lovers have problems with the nitty-gritty of having sex, simply because they have problems breaking through the hymen. This is the thin membrane of tissue that partly covers the entrance to the vagina. In some women this membrane is already torn, having been broken during strenuous activity as a child or by the insertion of tampons prior to even thinking about having sex. In many cases the hymen is, however, intact the first time you give sex a try. If your boyfriend feels he can't enter you or that something is blocking his way, this is the resistance of the hymen. If you feel a sharp pain and see some blood, this is the hymen breaking. The best way to help sex to happen is:

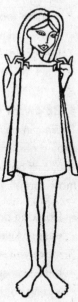

- To start off in the normal missionary position as this is the best one for first timers. Missionary is basically him on top of you, with both of you lying down.
- When he first penetrates you, push down with your vaginal muscles, as if you were about to pee.
- He should then thrust slowly and move deeper as you both relax and get into it.
- This will allow for your vagina to expand to accommodate him, and for the hymen to break allowing you finally to have sex.

2. Mention it's your first time

Virginity or sex for that matter does not put a neon sign over your head saying what you have or haven't done. As for 'Will he or won't he be able to tell?' 'Well, if your hymen's already broken (see above) the answer is 'No'. However, why lie? Having sex is a big deal and if you want it to be a good experience you can't go into it pretending you know everything there is to know.

3. Be kind if he's a virgin

There's always a first time for everyone. If you're about to have sex with someone who's a virgin, bear in mind that, unlike us females, male first timers need less foreplay. If you spend too long turning him on and bringing him to the brink of orgasm, he'll reach the point of no return and ejaculate before sex has even taken place. Your best bet therefore is to:

- Choose a position where you are in more control – perhaps on top, as this way you can pull away if he looks like he's coming too soon.
- Show him how you like to be touched and what makes you feel good, because this will be the stuff he won't know much about (unless of course you've been experimenting).

4. Be aware it might be painful

There can be a bit of pain as the hymen breaks. However, this should pass very quickly. If sex is still painful and he's inside you, or if he can't get inside you, the chances are you need more foreplay and need to take heed of the following:

- Don't be penetration obsessed. If you can't achieve it, it's easy to keep literally banging away at it; all this will do is make you sore and make penetration even less likely. You're better off spending more time on foreplay, oral sex and kissing so that you will relax first, and then try again.
- Try to relax. Subconsciously when we think something is going to hurt or be difficult we tense up, as a result the muscles in the vagina will clamp shut and act as a barrier.

Once this happens no amount of lubrication or force is going to do anything.

5. Timing is everything

Once you've both worked out how to turn each other on hugely, you'll not only know it in your mind but you should feel a ballooning feeling in your pelvic region, which will signal you are ready for penetration. Timing will also help in other areas, such as orgasm (see Chapter 4), so don't be surprised if the first time doesn't equal fireworks and sexual explosions. Like a first date, first-time sex can be a bit awkward and embarrassing. Don't let this be an indication of what's to come. Sex really does get better the more you do it.

6. Get your contraception sorted

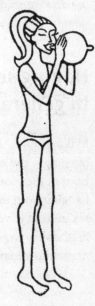

Contrary to popular opinion you can get pregnant the first time, even if he tries to use the withdrawal method. So unless you want to be one of the 110,000 UK girls who accidentally get pregnant each year, take precautions. You can also catch a sexually transmitted infection; so choose a method that also acts like a barrier i.e. a condom. (See Chapter 7 for more details on contraception.)

7. Don't be too adventurous too quickly

Master the basic sex positions before you start rolling and writhing like a whirling dervish on heat. You may be eager to experience the wilder side of sex, but it won't do much for you if you can't do the obvious bits. By all means don't just frolic in the missionary all night – get up, do it standing up, lean back, kiss him, tease him, feel him. Then when you're satiated, stop, have a rest and then wake him up later and go back in for more.

8. Don't expect too much

Good sex takes time and each time you have sex with someone new it can take a few goes to get it right. So if you don't have an orgasm, or found certain aspects unsatisfying and generally didn't have a good time, don't freak out. It doesn't mean you're useless at sex or frigid (horrible fake term that means nothing). It means you need to take more time with the simpler aspects of sex. Go back to the non-penetrative stage of sex and focus on kissing, foreplay and generally having a good time, then move towards sex again.

Having sex Part III – doing it in general

Making love, having sex, bonking, shagging, horizontal banging – the name of the game is endless, as are the variations of the moves. Luckily this is not the bit where I advocate hanging from the ceiling or going Tantric, or suggest you have sex in front of your neighbours. This is the bit where I suggest that variety in your technique is the key to sexual success, no matter how many times you've done it.

Successful sex

Variety in your sex life means:

- Variations in your foreplay technique.
- Changing positions.
- Experimenting with touch.
- Injecting some fun into your sex life.
- Thinking about quickies.
- Thinking about slowies.
- Telling him what he's doing right.
- Showing him what he's doing wrong.
- Asking for tips on how to improve your technique.
- Taking sex outside the bedroom.

The trouble with sex is, most of us meet someone, get loved up, have some pretty mind-blowing sexual adventures, and then sit back and settle down into a routine whereby sex becomes something to do on a rainy afternoon. After that most of us tend to live on sexual memories, reminding our partners of when we did that outrageous sex act or tried this, until one person gets bored and heads off to find someone who'll stop talking and start bonking.

This sad state of affairs happens because, like your route to work, if you take the same path every time you have sex, you move into autopilot mode. Which means you either start thinking about cleaning the kitchen floor when he's nuzzling your neck or start imagining you're with Brad Pitt.

So even if you have the sexual basics down to a fine art, for the sake of your enjoyment and your partner's it's always worth rebooting and extending your sexual repertoire. The good news is it's easier and takes less effort than you may think.

Sex positions

How many positions do you know? Three? Thirty? Three hundred? Whatever the number, think about how many you actually do and then why you do them. If the truth be known, you probably work your way around five and stick to them because: (1) they work, (2) you can do them, and (3) you're not one for wrapping your legs around your head. Fair enough – but you might like to know that you can vary most positions with just a small movement or simple bodily move, and turn something quite ordinary into a whole new sexual experience. Here's how:

1. The missionary

The most traditional sexual position, and, if surveys are to be believed, still the most popular. It may not be the most exciting but do it right and you not only get some good sex going but it also hits all the right buttons.

How to Do it:
You lie on your back with your legs apart, he lies on top of you and bingo – you have penetration.

How to Vary it:

- Do the above, but keep your legs closer together and straight as he penetrates, this will give you major clitoral stimulation.
- Alter the angle by wrapping your legs around his waist, also good for controlling his thrusts.

- Put a pillow under your bottom to tip you back for a deeper penetration.
- Get him to lie on top but move higher up your body so that he's resting on his arms and not squashing you. Then start thrusting slowly; his higher position will give you clitoral stimulation as he thrusts.

Good for: Intimacy, first-time sex, men who have trouble sustaining an erection. Especially good for the trigger-happy man who can't control ejaculation.

facts

The most prevalent position in the world for sex is the missionary position. In Italy it's known as the 'angelic position' and in the Middle East it's referred to as the 'manner of serpents'. For the majority of married people across the world it is used for 75 per cent of the sex they have.

2. Woman on top

As the name says – it's literally you on top of him. A favourite for most women as it allows them to take control of the situation and maintain a deep penetration. Men love it too because they don't have to do much. It's also a good way to control the depth of penetration, which helps if your partner's bits are on the large side. Also excellent if you're with a premature ejaculator as you can slow down if he looks like he's coming too soon.

How to Do it:

He lies out with his legs slightly apart; you climb abroad and straddle his hips, taking his penis inside you.

How to Vary it:

1. Lean forward to rub your clitoris against his pelvis area as you get into rhythm – this will pretty much guarantee an orgasm.

2. Lean towards his chest, tilting your pelvis to get a G-spot hit.

3. If you squat over him and lower down you can achieve very deep penetration.

4. Don't just thrust with him but move up and down to get the maximum effect of the position.

5. Finally try the position facing away from him, and lean forwards for extra depth.

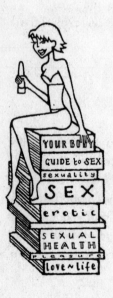

Good for: Women who want to take control of depth of penetration and thrusting speed. Also good for lazy men who want to have an easy ride, and excellent for clitoral stimulation during penetration.

3. Doggie position

This is sex from the behind as opposed to sex in the behind (see anal sex page 81) – so called because of the way dogs have sex. Men like this position because it feels naughty, gives them control over penetration and thrusting and allows them to go deep. Women like it because it often hits the G-spot, and gives the man easy access to her breasts, bottom and clitoris. On a down note, many women also find it painful because the depth of penetration means the head of the penis can sometimes connect painfully with the cervix.

How to Do it:
Get on your hands and knees, and with your boyfriend holding your hips from behind let him go for penetration.

How to Vary it:
1. Lower yourself down onto your elbows, this will change the depth of penetration.
2. Kneel against the side of the bed, resting your torso on the bed. This allows you to relax into the position, as you don't have to support yourself through his thrusts.
3. For those who feel extra strong and want an experimental edge try leaning over the bed and supporting your weight on your folded arms (put your head on a pillow). Your boyfriend should then come up to you in a standing position and lift your legs up to his waist and enter you from behind.

Good for: Deep penetration, making sex seem more naughty and for a G-spot hit.

"Positions and fancy moves are great, but there's nothing like having a close one on one simple session with someone you fancy the pants off."

Dan, 25

4. Standing

Good for a five-minute quickie, but not so great if there is a large difference between you in height and weight. Though it looks simple on film, the standing position is quite hard in reality as getting the angle of penetration right while standing often defies gravity and ruins the moment.

How to Do it:
You need to be at the right height for penetration, so this often means wrapping a leg around his waist.

How to Vary it:
1. Have your boyfriend literally lift you up and hold you.
2. If that's too hard, consider standing on something (not so sexy but it works).
3. Wear high heels – sexy and a way to use those shoes you can't bear walking in.

Good for: Couples who want to try something different and for intimacy and quickies.

facts

A study from Johns Hopkins University, USA, says having more sex is good for women as it raises levels of the female hormone oestrogen.

5. Side-by-side

This is a good position if you're looking for intimacy over loud rampant sex, as the movement is shallow and therefore limited. But it also has the advantage of lots of hands-on work alongside the sex.

How to Do it:
Lie side-by-side, literally, and rest your thigh over his leg for a better angle of penetration.

How to Vary it:
1. Move into spoons (he lies against your turned back) for a rear-entry side position.
2. Try bending your knees to wrap round him to allow greater depth of penetration in a face-to-face side-on move. Or bending them towards your waist in a spoons position.

Good for: Those who want to avoid deep penetration and for intimacy and slower sex.

6. Anal sex
Botty sex is not high on the majority of women's wish lists, as most women still consider it a taboo position and feel they'll be in pain/catch something nasty/and worst of all mess themselves up. Though that's not to say many women won't give it a try. According to the famous Kinsey Institute, USA, about 43 per cent of women have tried it, though less than 30 per cent of those found it pleasurable. It's a very high-risk activity (think HIV) so first up make sure you're well protected by using a strong condom. Also, make sure he goes slowly, as the anal tissues are very delicate and the anus is not elastic (unlike the vagina) so it can tear easily.

How to Do it:
Anal sex is painful for most women because relaxing the anal muscles is not easy. This is because there are two sphincters that need to be relaxed at the same time. A good way to

overcome this is to lubricate generously, then try to insert one finger for one minute, and bear down, which will relax both sphincters and help ease penile entry. Other tips include adopting the best position for rear entry:

1. On your back with a pillow under your hips. You can then put your arms under your thighs and lift them back to increase the curve and give him more access.
2. Or try sitting on top, and coming down over the penis.
3. Or a sex-from-behind position.

Good for: Those who feel like being a bit daring.

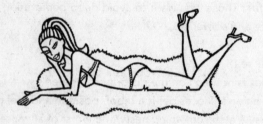

25 *ways*
to improve your sex life

1 Kiss Him
Sounds obvious but the biggest complaint from women about sex is that men forget to kiss them and just hone in on the sex zones. So take the initiative and go back to some heavy kissing – you won't be sorry, as researchers have found that kissing makes sex last longer, enhances orgasm, strengthens feelings of affection and boosts arousal.

2 Don't Gossip About Your Sex Life
Most men consider a sex revelation such as,'Goodness, does my boyfriend have a penis like a chipolata or what?' to be a major betrayal. If you want to continue reaping the benefits of his bedroom charms, keep quiet about your joint sexual exploits.

3 Minimise Distractions
Forget about what your mates are up to and don't think about how you're losing valuable drinking time. Contrary to popular opinion it's worth forgetting the annoying so-called ambience of music and candles too.

4 Turn Off The TV

Television has recently been voted the biggest libido killer. Watching TV in bed, apparently hypnotises you into wanting to sleep, desensitises you to sex and kills off your sex drive.

5 Control Yourself

Use your pelvic-floor muscles (the ones you use to pee with). Clench and release 20 times a day, and you'll soon be able to control your grip on his penis.

6 Play Hunt The G-spot

The elusive G-spot needn't be so elusive if you tell him what to look for. To find it, insert a finger into the vagina, move upwards and feel the front of the vaginal wall.

7 Try A Body-To-Body Massage

Get him to lie on his front and then lie on top of him. Now rub your body slowly up and down his; for an added boost you can slip your hand round to the front.

8 Don't Be Rough

Especially if you're exploring down below. He won't thank you if you yank and pull.

9 Get Oral With Him

If you're going down, do it right. Never make a face when you come up for air, don't hold your breath and never ever act as if you're doing him a huge favour.

10 Go Slow With The Oral

Behave like a woman dying of thirst at an oasis and you'll never bring him off. Start by using the flat of your tongue, rather than just the tip.

11 Bring A Banana To Bed

But not for the reason you're thinking. Bananas are a rich source of vitamin B and therefore eating them helps enhance both sex and orgasm by promoting the flow of blood to your sex organs.

12 Heat Things Up With Some Ice

Experts suggest keeping a cube in your mouth when you kiss, and when you're about to indulge in oral sex. Too cold to handle? Then try inserting a small cube into your vagina before penetration.

13 Steer Clear Of Household Objects

There are probably better ways to make your parents proud than inserting a Hoover part in your bottom (or his).

14 Be Selective About Food

Your vagina is not like your mouth, which means you can't just shove whatever you want in there and hope for the best. Certain foods (especially sugary ones) will aggravate the vaginal tissues. This means you could end up with some nasty lumps, bumps and itches.

15 Know His Penis Spots

The scrotal area, like the face, can easily become infected with little spots (especially as pubic hairs are curlier and can easily twist back into the follicle just like ingrown hairs on her bikini line). Occasionally, an infected follicle will form into a boil due to the warmth and humidity of the groin area.

16 Be Careful With His Bits

It's more than possible to injure an erect penis so be careful about how you throw yourself around the bed. If you hear a loud cracking noise, and you witness severe penile pain seek medical attention asap, as he's ruptured his penis and it needs to be splinted.

17 Don't Freak About No-Shows

Contrary to popular belief, erections are not under his voluntary control. This is why the commonest causes of erection problems are tiredness and stress. Statistics actually show that one man in seven (aged 16 and above) has erection problems at least four times a year.

18 Let Him Tie You Up

Good for control freaks who can't let go of being in charge. But remember this, the whole point of being the one tied up is that you can feign passivity and helplessness while all sorts of filthy, dirty things are done to you.

19 Forget The Average Sex Statistics

Ignore surveys or friends who claim they are having sex x-number of times a week. Sex is not a competition and it's what you get out of it, not how many times you have it, that counts.

20 Try The Scrotal Tug

No, this is not a rugby position but a prolonging technique that involves a gentle pull on the sac surrounding the testicles. Typically this extends arousal because it means a man can't ejaculate until the scrotum retracts and draws up close to his body. To perform a tug, gently hold the scrotal sac (just above the testicle) between your thumb and forefinger (make a ring shape) and pull gently downwards.

21 Experiment With Your No-Go Areas

Though sometimes scary, experimentation can improve your sex life by increasing your sexual confidence and helping push back your sexual boundaries. Try it if you dare (and want to) and then decide if it's for you or not.

22 Have Sex With Your Clothes On
Weird but true, one sex study showed that 64 per cent of women loved to fumble and grope with a half-clothed man.

23 Find Your Vaginal Cul-De-Sac
Believe it or not, just below the cervix is a highly sensitive passage, rich in nerve endings. This is known as the 'cul-de-sac'. Experts say if you clench your abdominal and PC muscles (the ones that control your pee flow), just as your boyfriend starts thrusting, you'll hit this area.

24 Never Mention Your Ex
Especially when you're both naked!

25 Don't Take Sex Too Seriously
It is meant to be fun you know!

CHAPTER FOUR

The orgasm stuff

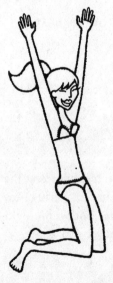

WHILE WE ALL HAVE THE PHYSICAL capacity to orgasm to our hearts' content, the truth is lots of women can't find one orgasm, never mind experience a multiple blast. The problem being, orgasms are frustratingly elusive. However, the good news for all lazy girls is, for once, trying harder won't actually help you achieve one. This is because to orgasm you need to be relaxed and if you're anxious, tense or pushing too hard, all that will happen is your orgasm will move further out of reach.

Though it may not feel like it, we actually have much better luck in the big O department than men. This is because men have what's biologically known as a refractory period – meaning they need a good old rest between their orgasms and the older they get, the longer that rest needs to be. Whereas once we find what works for us, we can actually fire orgasms off to our hearts' content. From a health and sex point of view, this is excellent news for the lazy girl because orgasms are full of health benefits.

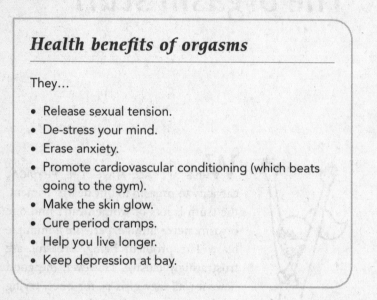

Health benefits of orgasms

They...

- Release sexual tension.
- De-stress your mind.
- Erase anxiety.
- Promote cardiovascular conditioning (which beats going to the gym).
- Make the skin glow.
- Cure period cramps.
- Help you live longer.
- Keep depression at bay.

Of course, the first step to orgasm is not in trying to beat the world record (134 if you're interested) but in discovering how you can help yourself achieve orgasmic bliss. Follow the right route and you too can have orgasms whenever you want.

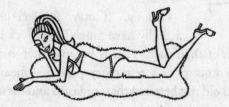

Orgasm basics

How to have an orgasm

The first rule of orgasms is to note that all orgasms vary. Not only from day to day, but from sensation to sensation, and from boyfriend to boyfriend. They also vary from woman to woman, which is why you may have heard stories about friends having to peel themselves off the ceiling, never really understanding how they got there in the first place. And that's the trouble with orgasms – people are just so competitive about them. So do yourself a favour and ignore tales of multiple orgasms and couples screaming the house down. While this may sound like something to aim for, it's not. Whatever your orgasm style it doesn't really matter because the pleasure comes from the fact you've had one, not your noise level.

Step one: *The arousal stage*
Relax and let go – easier said than done when all you want is to come, and fast. But getting tense, focusing on the outcome rather than the sex at hand and getting annoyed when you can't feel an orgasm happening will only deprive you of one. Instead of thinking about coming, think about what could turn you on because that's the key to getting on the orgasm road. Now add the following:

Physical stimuli: Think foreplay, oral sex, kissing, stroking each other, clitoral stimulation and naughty nothings whispered in your ear.

Emotional stimuli: Think mental turn-ons (see Chapter 2 for more ideas) and visual turn-ons i.e. his naked body, your body, scenarios that make you feel hot. Keep adding to the images in your mind while focusing on what you're doing to him and what he's doing to you.

facts

In Indianapolis, USA, oral sex is illegal even among married couples, and a similar law in Arizona, USA, says more than six women can't live together in the same house.

Signs of arousal

If you're aroused you should feel:

- Your nipples becoming erect.
- Your clitoris swelling.
- Your vagina lubricating (or getting wet).
- Your body heat rising.
- Increased blood flow to your genital region.

Step two: *Plateau*

This is the heightened version of the above. To get here you need to ensure you have continuous physical stimulation. Bear in mind if the stimulation stops you will go right back to the beginning and your boyfriend will have to start over.

Ways to keep it going: ensure he keeps up a steady rhythm

and tell him not to stop and start (a big male mistake with the female orgasm). Use your mental turn-ons to keep you going. Do not suddenly start thinking about the washing-up because, while this can help delay a man's orgasm, it will only plummet you back to base camp.

At plateau you should feel

- Super turned-on.
- On the brink of orgasm.
- A ballooning effect in your vagina as it lengthens and widens.

Step three: *The orgasm*
This is the peak of arousal and plateau – if nothing stops you here, you'll be free to pant your way to happiness through a succession of involuntary genital contractions, which should last anywhere from 10 to 60 seconds or longer.

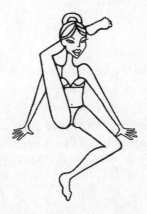

Yes, you're having an orgasm

- The body arches.
- Involuntary muscular contractions in your vagina and uterus – a bit like a pulsating sensation.
- Your pelvic and sphincter muscles tense up and your heart rate increases.
- Your nipples become erect and the areola will become slightly swollen.
- The clitoris becomes more engorged and starts to pull slightly.
- A slight flush may spread across your breasts.
- Your breathing escalates.
- Release occurs and you'll feel vaginal, pelvic and even anal contractions, which will increase to one every 0.8 seconds.
- You'll feel as if all the sexual tension in your body has been sucked out.
- You feel elated, satiated, relieved.

Step four: *Resolution*

This is back to square one. However, if your boyfriend carries on with stimulation you can go back to plateau and have another orgasm. If not, your body will go back to normal. Don't freak if nothing happened after the plateau stage. Orgasms, like most things in life, depend on your mood and the way you go about getting them; meaning each time will be different for you.

Different types of orgasm

Okay, now you've found your orgasm (hopefully) here's where it gets a tad complicated because there is in fact more than one type of orgasm. Before you run screaming from the bedroom, bear in mind this is a very good thing. Apart from meaning you'll now have to experiment more, it also means you have a whole host of ways of reaching sexual nirvana.

The clitoral orgasm

This is by far the most common type of orgasm, as it results from directly stimulating the clitoris and surrounding area of the vagina (for more tips go to Chapters 2 and 3).

Clitoral orgasms are usually the first type of orgasm you'll ever experience and the ones that are most likely to happen on your solo and joint ventures. The good thing about them is they can easily be achieved during penetration with various positions aiding stimulation, or with some hands-on help (see page 101).

This type of orgasm packs a punch due to the make-up of the clitoris.

New findings by Australian scientists in the *Journal of Urology* have recently highlighted the fact that the clitoris is attached to an inner mound of erectile tissue which extends about 11cm (4.25in) inside your body. This and the surrounding muscle tissues all contribute towards the powerful muscle spasms that make up an orgasm.

The vaginal orgasm

This is a more elusive orgasm – some women can get them at a drop of a hat, others have more problems. They occur when the inner walls of the vagina and/or the G-spot (the mass of spongy tissue found on the front wall of your vagina) are stimulated through intercourse or with fingers. The G-spot is especially effective as it swells when stimulated.

To find the G-spot during sex:

- Lie on your back and tilt your pelvis upwards so that your vulva presses against your boyfriend's pelvic bone, this should make for direct contact on the G-spot with penetration.
- If you still can't find it put some pillows under your bottom, to increase the angle.

"What's with men and all that thrusting? I wish guys would realise it's not sexy, it doesn't help us to come and all it does is make us pretty desperate to throw a fake one just so you'll stop."

Sarah, 25

The multiple orgasm

Studies show that fewer than 30 per cent of women experience multiple orgasms. This could either be a fact or a sign that some women don't realise they are having multiples when they are. Unlike the movies, when you see women wracked by a series of amazingly active orgasms, multiples in real life tend to be smaller and spaced a few seconds or sometimes a few minutes apart. They can be achieved by literally carrying on with stimulation after the first orgasm has passed. However, don't be too focused on the multiple sensation. If you're keen to have more than one orgasm during sex, it's easier to go for one during foreplay, another during sex and/or oral sex, etc. If you can never find more than one, don't feel disappointed – like everything in life it's quality not quantity that counts in the end.

The simultaneous orgasm

Studies show the chances of reaching peak at the same time as your bloke are fairly low, especially if your bodies are different sizes and you don't know each other's major hot spots. The main problem is: we take longer to build to the pre-orgasmic phase; meaning that though we are in the same race, he'll be over the finish line quaffing the champagne, while we're still warming up. However, the simultaneous O can be achieved and here's how.

Step one: *Go for joint arousal*
The first trick is to get your sexual responses in sync, which means getting to the same level of arousal. One slight flick of the hand will probably get him from 0 to 100 in two seconds,

so the aim of his game is to delay penetration and ejaculation for as long as possible.

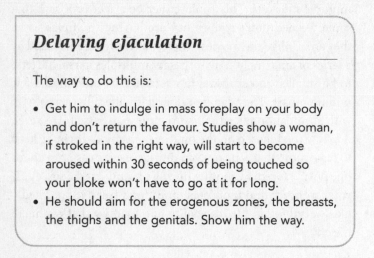

Delaying ejaculation

The way to do this is:

- Get him to indulge in mass foreplay on your body and don't return the favour. Studies show a woman, if stroked in the right way, will start to become aroused within 30 seconds of being touched so your bloke won't have to go at it for long.
- He should aim for the erogenous zones, the breasts, the thighs and the genitals. Show him the way.

Step two: *Make sure he does his job*

To sustain arousal, make sure your guy keeps up his end of the bargain and works on physical stimulation (remember you can help him out if he gets tired or runs out of ideas). Also have a swift look at him. If at any stage you see the head of his penis enlarge and his testicles draws closer to the body, give up your chances of a mutual climax and go for penetration because this is a sign he's about to come.

If he can hold off (tell him to think about something dull), look for signs that you're approaching orgasm so you're ready to go to the next stage. Your muscles will also start to tense all over your body and lubrication will increase.

If you can feel all this – you're ready to go for it.

facts

Rare individuals: 1 in every 1,250 men can orgasm instantly by concentrating on sexual fantasies without any genital manipulation. As for erection speed, while this is determined by factors such as fitness, fatigue and age, a few remarkable men can achieve full erection in as little as three seconds.

Step three: *Get your pace in sync*
The second your pelvic muscles tense up (you'll feel a tightening sensation in your pelvic floor and your bottom) go for penetration. The aim is now to get your pace in sync.

If you try the CAT (Coital Alignment Technique, see page 101) position, his pelvic bone will rub the clitoris as he thrusts, adding to the sensation. If you can build from here at an equal and steady pace, the likelihood that you'll finally come together is pretty much assured.

Orgasm benefits and lies

The benefits

- It will boost your mood. According to a study from the University of Virginia, USA, orgasms boost levels of oestrogen, which in turn makes you feel happier.
- It will increase intimacy, as oxytocin (the hormone that helps you bond with someone) goes to five times its normal level during orgasm.

- It will make you feel relaxed – a study in the *Journal of the American Medical Association* shows that 20 minutes of sex triggers a two-hour relaxation response.
- Cures insomnia – orgasm induces the sleep hormone, which means 20–30 minutes after climax you'll be in the land of nod.
- Gives you a healthy heart – three orgasms a week reduce your risk of heart disease by 50 per cent.
- It will keep you young and healthy – have orgasms twice a week and you'll avoid colds and strengthen your immune system.

The lies

1. Orgasms can go on for hours.
Reality: sadly (or rather, thankfully) not. The typical male orgasm lasts from 6 to 10 seconds and the typical female orgasm lasts from 10 to 60 seconds.

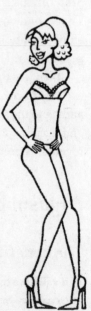

2. There's only one way to orgasm
Reality: there are at least six different types of female orgasm – clitoral, vaginal, G-spot, multiple, simultaneous and fantasy (on your own), all of which bring different intensities to the results.

3. Sex is useless, unless you reach an orgasm
Reality: if this was true, hardly any women would bother having penetrative sex, as studies show only 30 per cent of females orgasm during intercourse alone.

4. Men always orgasm

Also untrue. If a guy's tired he may be able to maintain an erection but won't orgasm or ejaculate (male orgasm is the feeling men get with ejaculation, they are not the same thing).

5. Women often pee on orgasm

Reality: the fluid release is not pee but something known as female ejaculation. Still worried,well don't be: the Kinsey Institute on Sex, USA, found that as many as 40 per cent of women had experienced at least one ejaculation at orgasm.

Best lazy girl ways to have orgasms

The list is endless, but to save you from becoming an orgasm geek, here are the four best moves to ensure you have the best sex of your life.

CAT

The Coital Alignment Technique (CAT), otherwise known as perfecting the angle of his dangle during the missionary.

Most women don't achieve orgasm from penetration alone, so the trick is to get your clitoris in on the act. The theory behind the well-known CAT position is simple:

- He gets on top of you and lines up his pelvis over yours. This means he lies higher up your body than usual, resting on elbows so that when he enters you he's riding high. This means he will then press against your pubic bone and clitoris as he thrusts.
- For extra pressure he could lie his full weight on you (do not attempt if he is much, much bigger than you are) and then you should wrap your legs around his thighs.

- You then push up with your pelvis as he pushes down. If you press against each other as you do it and keep your pace steady, an orgasm will be guaranteed.

G-spotting

The elusive G-spot is, say the sexperts, directly connected to the orgasm core in the brain, which is why it's such a well-known pleasure centre. Though many people speculate on whether the G-spot (named after Dr Ernst Grafenburg) even exits, many women who have found the spot report deeper, longer and more intense orgasms. If you want to experience the G-spot sensation, it's worth noting you can only feel the G-spot when you're aroused, as this is when the area swells with blood and becomes raised.

It can then be found 5cm (2in) into your vagina, on the front wall.

G-spot orgasm

A good way to stimulate the G-spot during sex is to go for the old sex-on-a-table routine.

- Lie down with your back completely straight.
- Now when your bloke comes up, hook your legs over his shoulders and get him to hold on to your hips as he enters you.
- Once he starts thrusting, his penis will firmly hit your G-spot area.
- When this first happens you may feel like you need to pee (the G-spot is near your urethra) but this sensation will decrease and soon an orgasmic feeling will take over.

The PC clench

We all have love muscles, which are known as the PC (pubo-coccygeal) muscles. In women they control the size and grip of the vagina, which is why it's essential to get them working. If you tone these muscles you can enhance your orgasms, and make them so powerful you can cause your boyfriend to come.

To build them up all you have to do is stop the flow of pee, when you're on the loo, for 10 to 15 seconds and release. Do it regularly and you'll boost your sex life tenfold.

The best position for testing those muscles is the woman on top. Climb aboard and straddle your bloke.

Make sure your weight is distributed evenly between both legs, and, on penetration, try moving in small circles as you lift up and down.

When he can't bear the teasing any longer, bear down and clench your PC muscles (slowly at first in case they are super strong) so he can feel you gripping him. At the same time get him to make good use of his hands (focusing on the breasts and clitoris), and lie back and let go.

facts

Forty-four per cent of Brazilian women confess to faking orgasm. Forty-nine per cent of UK women have trouble reaching an orgasm.

The back bend

(Variation on seated sex/woman on top)

- Have your bloke sit in a sturdy chair and climb onto his lap.
- Now hook your thighs over his, and slowly lean back.
- The aim is to practically lie on his lap and let your head and shoulders hang off the edge of his knees (he does all the supporting).
- If you feel unsafe, put your arms behind your head so you can touch the ground.
- You should then hold his hips and literally pull yourself towards him, and he enters you. For an extra buzz arch your back and pelvis upwards as he thrusts.

The plunge

(Variation on missionary)

Slowly lie backwards, resting first on your hands and then elbows and then all the way down so that eventually you're lying flat with your thighs open and legs folded underneath you.

Now throw your arms above your head, get him to lie on top of you and enter you.

The trick is not to move so that the angle of the plunge will give you a deep and satisfying penetration (all thanks to the fact your knees have elevated your pelvis).

Against the wall

(Variation on standing and doggie position)

Face your bedroom wall and bend so outstretched arms are resting on the wall.

- Your legs should be apart and your bottom sticking out in the air.
- Now get him to come up behind you, lean his body over hold onto your hips and enter you from behind.
- At the same get him to move his hands round to your clitoris for extra stimulation.
- This works particularly well if you have a large height variation and can't manage sex face to face standing up.

The quickie

Perfect for those who slack on the detail and can't be bothered to get undressed properly. The quickie gets a bad press but really can be just as hot and satisfying as a long drawn-out session as long as it's not the norm. The good news is you can do it anywhere (just pull your knickers aside), it stops the rot of sex in bed at the regular weekly time, and it's thrilling.

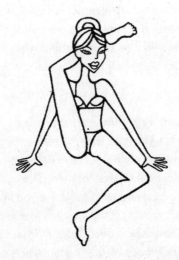

Troubleshooting

1. I can't have an orgasm during sex, only when I'm alone

Sex can be a very anxiety-ridden venture especially if you're having sex with someone you really like, or someone you don't know very well. This anxiety unfortunately works against orgasms, which are about the release of sexual tension through letting go (something you can't do when you're anxious).

To get the orgasm you want all you need to do is communicate the technique that works best for you when you're alone. For instance: manual stimulation, fantasy, oral sex or a fast/slow/steady rhythm. Remember, as you can already orgasm on your own, you can definitely have one when you're with a guy by showing him the way. All you have to do is feel more confident about saying what you want in bed and relax about whether or not it's going to happen. To feel braver, try extending the time spent on foreplay as this will: (1) make you feel less anxious about what comes after, and (2) take your mind away from the fear that orgasm won't happen again.

2. I don't orgasm every time we have sex

Most women don't. The idea that the female orgasm naturally occurs every time you have sex is a male notion simply because this is how it happens for men. The best way to orgasm is to lead his hand right to where you like to be touched and start moving it the way you like to be stimulated after the penetrative sex is over. The aim is let him know loud and clear that sex is not over just because he's come.

"My ex-boyfriend was so hung up on how many times I orgasmed during sex. It got to the stage where I felt I was in this race and if I didn't score more than one I'd let him down."

Sue, 23

3. He takes ages to come

If your man's all thrust and no lift off, you're not alone. Many men have the bizarre notion that women love vigorous amounts of thrusting because they don't understand how the female anatomy works. As we know – the part of our body which is the most sexually sensitive is the clitoris and this gets no hit whatsoever from thrusting into a nerve-free vagina. If your boyfriend doesn't understand this, and you're raw from waiting for him to come, try highlighting his wrongdoings by showing him the power of a simple clitoral touch, i.e. place his hand on the spot. At the same time, swap positions. An on-top position will have you controlling the pace, and speed; meaning he won't be able to go for a marathon thrust session, and you'll be able to make him wait until you're ready to come.

4. He doesn't notice I fake it

It's likely he doesn't notice because women fake so often, most men have no idea what a real orgasm looks like. Plus it's likely you have timed it to coincide with his orgasm, which is when he's least likely to notice the roof falling in, never mind your climax. The real question to ask yourself is why aren't you being honest? Whatever your reason, you need to let him know asap that sex isn't working for you. The best way to do this is to show him what turns you on. Show him how you like to be touched, and then tell him with loud moans and groans how it feels.

5. I can't orgasm at all

For many, the road to 30 seconds or more of pleasure is one littered with psychological roadblocks. The big problem is, and here comes the science, the more you panic about not having an orgasm, the more stress chemicals from your brain are released. These send anxiety waves coursing through your body and push the chance of an orgasm even further away. Help yourself by practising on your own (for more tips see Chapter 2). Pick a quiet location, the bathroom, a locked bedroom, watch something that turns you on, or read something erotic. Then let your hands slip and slide over your body until you feel yourself getting close and letting go.

6. He faked it

With condoms it's not always easy to tell if your boyfriend's come or not. The fact is men sometimes fake it too, usually because they are tired and rarely because they don't fancy you. If you suspect he's not telling you the truth don't make a big deal of it. The chances are he's faking it because he's freaked and also because he doesn't want to hurt your feelings.

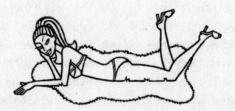

25 ways
to orgasm

1 Read Something Sexy
Don't think words aren't sexy. The women's erotica market (i.e. porn stories aimed at women) has thrived considerably of late. Check out a raunchy novel and see how quickly it fires you up.

2 Exercise Three Times A Week
It will not only improve your sex drive and your flabby bits but also boost your orgasms, as you'll have more stamina and more strength to keep going for longer.

3 Have Sex In The Morning
Your hormone levels and sex drive will be in sync with his and so your chances of orgasm are much higher than late at night.

4 Know Your Monthly Hormonal Highs
It will help you to get the best out of your sex life.
Tip: days 7–14 are best for orgasm, though it does depend on the woman. Some of you might find pre-period days are your most orgasmic.

5 Pay Attention To What You're Doing

Forget about how you need to do some laundry, or how you're missing your favourite soap; paying attention to your body and staying connected to what's happening to you will improve your orgasm in an instant.

6 Do Your Pelvic Floor Exercises

Clench and release your PC muscle 20 times a day (this is the muscle you pee with). You'll improve your orgasms and his, as you'll have stronger contractions during your orgasm, and also be able to grip him more during penetrative sex.

7 Find Both Your G-Spots

Yours is on the front of the internal vaginal wall (only look when you're aroused, otherwise you won't find it), his is located on the front rectal wall (i.e. up his bottom).

8 Ask For More Oral

It's a lie that men don't like it and it's a guaranteed way to orgasm.

9 Go Slow With Your Oral Technique

Slowly but firmly is the key and then build up your speed. Do it right and he'll be buying you presents for the rest of the year.

10 Improve The Missionary Position

For better clitoral stimulation keep your legs straight

and close together while he's thrusting so you have a stronger chance of orgasm during sex.

11 Get On Top More
It will allow you to control the speed and depth of penetration – which is good for your orgasms, as you get to say when he comes. (If he looks like he's coming too soon, lift off him and move down only when he's moved back a phase.)

12 Ignore The Sex Myths
Remember, if it sounds unlikely, it is unlikely, especially when it comes to orgasms.

13 Be Imaginative
Not just about positions, but also about locations, clothing and what you're thinking as your having sex together.

14 Be Firm About What You Want
Believe it or not, 85 per cent of men say it's sexy to have sex with a woman who knows what she wants in bed. This is good news because it means you'll get what you need to orgasm and he'll be super turned on.

15 Let Him Know Less Is More
Banging away in the same position is boring and painful and not the way to orgasm – tell him now before he ruins your sex life.

16 Make Him Last Longer

It will make your orgasm more likely. To help him achieve this, get him to focus on you and extend his staying power by not touching him until the last possible moment.

17 Don't Fret About Your Wobbly Bits

Contrary to popular opinion, men don't equate hot sex with the body of model, and if you're too focused on holding your stomach in you will never orgasm during sex.

18 Slow Your breathing Down

As in slow your breathing down as you approach orgasm. Most of us breathe more quickly as we feel ourselves peaking and tense up trying to bring the orgasm on. If instead you relax your tummy, and take slow, deep breaths into your stomach, the orgasm will not only last longer, it will also be more intense.

19 Don't Be Orgasm Obsessed

Bizarrely stress yourself out about achieving nirvana and you'll never reach it.

20 Laugh More

It will help you relax during sex and make your orgasms more likely.

21 Touch Yourself

His hands can't be everywhere at once, so if he's at your breasts or stroking your back, move your own hands down and do what needs to be done.

22 Watch A Dirty Movie

Okay, you may not think you'll be turned on by something visual, but forget porn and think about your favourite sex scene from a movie or your favourite actor getting down to it. Switch it on and imagine it's happening to you – it will get you to climax faster than you think.

23 Go Tantric

Practise Tantric sex (two hours of foreplay and then no thrusting during penetration) and rather than just feeling an orgasm in your genital region you'll experience an all over body climax.

24 Fake It To Make It

After saying faking was a no-no, there is an American theory that claims if you start faking that you're having an orgasm, i.e. start breathing rapidly, then try to contract your vaginal muscles you'll actually end up having an orgasm.

25 Give Each Other A Sensual Massage

Corny, but it works – especially if you do it slowly and with oil!

CHAPTER FIVE

The problematic stuff

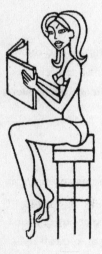

So YOU'VE HAD SEX, you've had an orgasm, you've kissed and licked and basically hoovered your way around his body. Perhaps, you've had three orgasms in a row, a simultaneous and then went back in for more. If so, good for you, but while I don't want to be the one to throw a wet blanket over your passionate lovemaking, it's worth bearing in mind that even the most dynamic sexual relationship can go through the odd hiccup now and again. Which is why learning to ask the right questions about sex and knowing how to respond is the key to maintaining a happy and exciting sex life.

Good questions to ask about your sex life

1. Is this position good for me?

Why you should ask this: There are positions that can aid your orgasm, positions that make sex more intimate and positions that make sex wilder and naughtier than you could ever have imagined. Then, sadly there are plain stupid positions, ones that hurt like hell, and ones that do absolutely nothing for either of you. Of course, to find the right moves for your relative sizes and desires it's usually a case of test-driving a number of different positions. However, things to remember when considering a move are:

- If it's painful it's not worth doing.
- If it makes you feel uncomfortable (both mentally and physically) you don't have to do it.
- And finally, if it concertinas your stomach, your best bet is to turn the light off first.

2. Do I really want to do this?

Why you should ask this: We all want to be seen as wild and adventurous vixens in bed, and while this can lead you down the path of bizarre, wonderful and mind-blowing sex (see Chapter 6), it can also lead you to potential embarrassment and regret. So before you attempt anything ask yourself the above question and be really honest about your answer. Areas to think twice about are:

- Sex in your office because, let's face it, you will end up on a security camera.

- Sex in a public place. Yes, it's still an offence to be caught having sex where others and small children can see you.
- Sex in a dangerous place. Remember sex should be dangerous as in exciting, not dangerous as in potentially life-threatening.
- Sex that could hurt too much, this includes S&M, anal sex and any kind of bizarre role-playing that equals more pain than you think you can handle.
- Sex that you won't be able to live with afterwards: this is a threesome with your best mate, naked pictures and a live webcam.
- Sex with your boss or a married man – need we go here?

3. Am I doing the right thing?

Why you should ask this: In a US sex survey 85 per cent of women said they couldn't tell if their bloke was enjoying sex with them or not. So here are a few tips: if your hand and brain's gone numb you should probably stop doing what you're doing and check if he's still awake. If he looks like he's moaning in pain, rather than ecstasy you should also stop immediately, and finally, if he keeps pushing your hands in a particular direction, you should probably go with the flow because he's trying to tell you something.

If any or all of the above sound familiar, it's time to ask him outright what he'd like you to do because this will not only help your sex life, make you feel more confident and generally improve your relationship, but also make him feel massively turned on.

Signs your man's enjoying it

If you're dating a non-verbal type, body-language signals to watch out for are:

- The right kind of groans and yelps.
- Dilated pupils.
- A rosy flush across his bottom and genitals.

4. Am I being too scary?

Why you should ask this: If you've already reached the borders of depravity and it's your first date, then it's likely you are being more than a bit scary. While most blokes like the idea of wild sex, most live in fear that the women they're with will turn bonkers, especially when naked. Hints that you're being scary are:

- Your boyfriend attempts to avoid sex at all costs.
- There is blind terror in his eyes every time you get into the bedroom.
- He feebly suggests that you just do it normally tonight.

If you want to get hot and wild, then there are ways to introduce it slowly into your sex life (see Chapter 6). So start with suggestions for mild wildness, like blindfolding, light S&M, and gentle role-play. Then as his courage increases, you can introduce more and more elements, so you don't freak him out. Ultimately, even though a bit of naughtiness will heighten intimacy, there are a few basics you should agree to before you begin:

- Always best to decide how far you both will go before you start.
- Choose a word or phrase that you can use that will make you or him stop immediately.
- Don't push him if he says 'No'!

Questions not to ask about sex

Tempting to ask, but disastrous to use:

1. Am I better at sex than your ex?

If you're even bothering to ask this question, then it's likely you're not going to believe his answer. The fact is we all feel insecure about sex, and more so if his last girlfriend happened to look like a supermodel. However, no amount of reassurance that you're more of a sex goddess than her will make you feel better. If you can't fathom the fact he's dating you, not her, you need to boost your self-esteem, not beg for compliments.

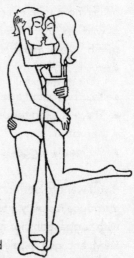

2. Is that it?

If you've been left lacking in the sexual highs department, there are better ways to get more out of your boyfriend than humiliating him into a response.

Start by showing him the way (literally), and making the right noises when he hits the spot. Loud ohs and yeses usually mark the way pretty clearly even for the dimmest of men.

"I'm not that big down below and some women are pretty nasty about it. One girl just went on and on about how she couldn't feel anything and how I was tiny and maybe should see a doctor. It left me feeling really self-conscious about sex for a long time."

Perry, 24

3. Is it in yet?

We all know that men are pretty sensitive about the size of their willies, so don't make him feel worse if he's not blessed with an average-sized penis (and let's face it some men aren't). If you can't resist, imagine how you'd feel if he looked into your bra and said, 'Mmm... is that it?'

Not getting any satisfaction? Well think about other ways to improve your sex life, more oral, more foreplay and a different position, such as a behind entry, can all help.

4. Can you tell if I'm faking or not?

Okay, you may be joking but all this is really going to do is send him the message that you may have faked prior to this comment, you will fake in the future, and that he's so crap at sex you obviously have to fake!

If your aim is to turn him into an insecure, bumbling wreck then you're going about it the right way. If you're just kidding – don't!

Top 8 female sexual worries

Worried, anxious, stressed about sex? If so, it's likely you're grappling with a very common and easily solvable sex problem. Take a look at the following and find the lazy way to make sex easier for yourself.

1. I'm too dry during sex

Some women find they are literally overflowing in the lubrication department, while others find they always need a little help. It's not a sign you're not sexed-up enough or there's something amiss in your sexual make-up, but just the way your body works. To help yourself along, and avoid painful sex, all you need to do is introduce some KY jelly into the proceedings. The joy of KY is it's odour free, painless to buy and water-based so it won't eat away at your condom. At the same time, slow sex down, add more foreplay into the mix and don't attempt penetration until you are lubricated.

Lazy solution: Use KY and take your time over foreplay.

facts

Think all that body rubbing is a load of new age non-sense? Well think again. New studies show rubbing, kissing, stroking and/or petting an erogenous zone is the fast track to good sex. It seems one simple touch will cause sexual messages to race to his brain at the speed of around 260kph (160mph). Keep it going and you could have his body on fire and aching for you in just over three minutes.

2. My vagina makes noises like I am breaking wind when I have sex

Sex is sometimes a downright embarrassing business and, as many girls know, that windy, loud air-expelling whoosh during sex is perhaps the most embarrassing aspect of all. It happens because when a man penetrates you so does a fair amount of air, which means at some point or another, the air has to exit your body, hence the embarrassing fart-like sound effects. Changing position can help reduce the noise, as certain manoeuvres like doggy position, legs on his shoulders, etc. make it more likely to happen. The least noisy position is the missionary, but seeing as you can't have sex this way for ever, just relax and make a joke about what's happening.

Lazy solution: Laugh it off.

3. My boyfriend's boring in bed

Are you with someone who thinks exciting sex means sex twice in one night? Does the hint of sexual experimentation have him running for cover? It sounds simple but the first step here to is to speak up. Good sex can only happen if you let each other know through words, actions and experimentation what's working and what's not. If you're not speaking up, ask yourself why? Is it because you're afraid he'll think you're slutty or weird? If so try something new but simple, jump on top of him, say something naughty or simply rev up the speed.

Lazy solution: Try something new.

4. Our sex drives are out of sync

Okay so he's not on for full sex every night of the week; well, it's a myth that men always want and are ready for sex. The libido varies, and just as a woman can have a low sex drive so too can a man. So stop imagining his lack of interest is about you. Lack of libido can be about anything from too much alcohol to stress at work and tiredness. Then think about ways you can both compromise on your sex drives. Perhaps, think of non-penetrative ways of having sex, including oral sex and simple foreplay to orgasm. This way you can be satiated and he can get to sleep early.

Lazy solution: Compromise on what you want.

5. I hate my body
Unless you have the physique of a model it's likely there's something about your body parts that you just don't like. If so don't obsess about it. Everyone (even men) worry their body is not ravishing enough, their technique not expert enough, or their bits not big/small/firm enough. Dangerous thinking because if you can't accept your body the way it is you will

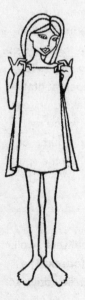

never believe someone who says they find you attractive. Instead focus on your positive points (and, yes, we all have at least one). Finally, think about what you're doing to your boyfriend. No one likes to have to reassure someone all the time. It's insulting, not to mention exhausting.

Lazy solution: Stop looking at yourself.

6. Sex gets boring with the same person
Boredom in bed is a common female complaint, and yet very few women do anything about it. The fact is, there are plenty of ways to keep sex interesting, but they involve both of you trying new things, not

"A girl who I saw sucked her stomach in throughout sex and refused to go on top because she said I'd see her double chin. It's a huge turn-off when girls act like this."

Seb, 26

you waiting for your boyfriend to introduce a new move. Unsure if you can go for it? Well, studies show that being proactive during sex equals a more satisfying sex life, more orgasms, more confidence and a relationship that lasts longer than most.

Lazy solution: Try harder.

7. You feel too big for him

Some women's vaginas are just built bigger than others are, in the same way some men hang larger than their friends. If you find you're too big to 'grip' his penis, here's how to make sex more pleasurable.

- Do your PC workout every day. These are a series of exercises called Kegels (developed in the 1950s) designed to strengthen the pelvic-floor muscles, which contract during orgasm to give you that pulsating feeling.With strong PCs you can grip anything.
- Step one is to locate your PC muscle. Do this by stopping your pee midway and holding for a count of five and releasing.
- Step two is to contract and relax the muscle without holding it, 25 times, twice a day. Start off slowly and then

build up your reps and do them as fast as you can. Finally work up to 50 and hold each one for a count of three.

- When you're having sex, alter your position so your vagina seems tighter. The best way to do this is to go for a rear-entry position, or lift your pelvis when he enters you. Also keep your legs close together as this will keep the angle of your vagina tight and narrow and allow you more feeling during sex.

- Finally get on top and lean back. When he penetrates, this will alter the slant of the vagina and make you feel smaller inside to him, plus it will increase the friction, upping your chances of orgasm.

Lazy solution: Do a vaginal workout.

8. I'm too tight for sex

If you think you're small in the front-bottom department, here's how to solve it.

- Choose a position that goes for less penetration, i.e. missionary or woman on top, rather than doggy. This will allow you to have more control of depth and speed of penetration.

- Make sure you're well lubricated. Often tightness is really lack of moisture, and adding lubrication (such as KY jelly) can make sex not only more comfortable, but totally painless too.

- Don't push – you need to expand widthways as well as get lubed up. So wait for that ballooning feeling before going for penetration.

- Ban quickies. Give yourself time to get turned on – as foreplay will allow your vagina time to expand in order to accommodate him.

facts

Twenty per cent of French people say they have no interest in sex.

- Make penetration easier by bending your knees and spreading your legs as he moves inside you. Also try dropping your tailbone as he enters, as this gives him an easier entry angle and helps loosen vaginal muscles.
- Finally make sure he goes slowly. This way you won't clench your vaginal muscles in anticipation of pain. Make him enter, then pull back until you're completely ready for full penetration.

Lazy solution: Change positions.

Top four male sexual hitches

(And what you can do about them.)
Okay, they may be his problem but they'll be yours too especially if you don't work on ironing them out. Like female glitches, male sexual hitches are easily fixed.

1. He can't get it up
Not as unusual as you think, and it rarely has anything to do with you, but before you reach for the Viagra, consider his lifestyle:

- If he's a couch potato who survives on pizza, beer and cigarettes, his erection rate will be lower than most. Factors such as stress also play a major role in no-shows. If it's a recurring problem, check his stress levels: exam pressure, unemployment, family problems and work hassle will all affect his ability in bed. If this is behind his no-shows, he needs to work out how to reduce the pressure in his life.

- Ninety-seven per cent of men have at least one no-show (or more) a year and the main culprit is too much booze. If your boyfriend has been drinking all night, the chances of him being able to get it up, never mind sustain erection, are low to zero.

- Fatigue is also a reason why guys can't get it up. Unlike women, men need lots of energy to get blood pumping to the penis. If he's tired, don't force him to go at it, wait until the morning when he'll be rejuvenated and on a testosterone high.

- Finally, remember, if your bloke wakes up with an erection or can get one during masturbation, his problem is not medical but psychological.

2. He comes too soon

Premature ejaculation, also known as coming too soon, is also fairly common in men in their early twenties. It happens to guys who haven't learnt to control and extend the plateau phase, which occurs just prior to orgasm. This is usually the result of their masturbation technique, i.e. doing it too fast. The good news is this means it can be changed with a little help from you:

- Give the stop/start technique a try. Which basically means you start to have sex, then stop and completely withdraw the minute you feel he is about to come. Stop stimulation completely until he loses his erection and then repeat three times before allowing him to ejaculate. Sex therapists say this is 90 per cent effective if you keep practising it.

- Another technique is called the squeeze. This is where you apply pressure just below the head of the penis before a guy is about to come. You need to apply pressure for at least four seconds with the pads of your fingers.
- In terms of your enjoyment – getting him to give you an orgasm before sex can help leave you less frustrated until he masters control.
- Also suggest he tries distraction techniques if he feels he's about to come, such as thinking about his granny or keeping his eyes shut, so he can't be visually stimulated by your luscious body.
- Lastly, try keeping still for a while. It sounds boring but lying still and not throwing yourself into sex can delay ejaculation so sex lasts a bit longer until he learns control.

3. He's too small

Size matters, but rarely in the way a man thinks. Width, rather than length can make all the difference during penetration simply because all the most sensitive nerve endings of the vagina are near the front, which means an immediate pleasure hit when this area is stretched, or when pressure is applied to it.When a penis is narrow or too small, a lot of this satisfaction is missed, especially during the thrusting stage of intercourse. However, with a bit of manoeuvring you can improve the situation.

- Firstly start by placing a pillow under your hips so your pelvis tilts backwards allowing for possible G-spot stimulation on the front wall of your vagina.

- Clenching your PC muscles (the ones you use when you pee) can also help grip him as he starts pumping, giving you the sensation you need.
- Finally, if none of the above work, sit on him. An upright lap position can help you to control not only the action but also enable you to move about on top of him so you can get the right feeling as he penetrates.

4. He's too big

If your boyfriend's penis is on the large side it's likely the positions that allow for deeper penetration are not right for you. Being on top and having sex from behind make it more likely that his penis will hit the cervix, which in turn will equal pain, as the area is full of nerve endings. Your best bet is to use the positions that make sex comfortable for you.

- Besides the missionary, try a side-by-side entry, which is shallower, or a variation on the woman on top.

"Size matters for us girls. One guy I know dropped his pants and I nearly fainted because he was so wide in the willy department. I had to make every excuse under the sun to avoid penetration because the thought of that coming anywhere near me made my eyes water."

Abby, 22

- Instead of letting him guide your hips down onto him in this position, make him lie back and let you take complete control over the depth of penetration. Proceed slowly with entry and lift yourself off if you start to feel uncomfortable.
- The aim is to eventually find the right spot – a place where penetration feels highly pleasurable, not painful. If the pain doesn't go away or spreads, go for a sexual health check-up at your nearest GUM clinic to make sure a hidden STI isn't the problem (see Chapter 7).
- If he can't get it in, don't hammer away at it – this will just make your vagina tense up even more. Instead get him to pull out and up the foreplay.With width issues you need the vagina to expand as well as lengthen, when this occurs you'll feel a ballooning feeling in your vagina and this should signal you're now ready for penetration.

Post-sex loving

What's the first thing that happens after sex? Do you kiss, cuddle, talk for hours, or kick your boyfriend in the ribs as he starts snoring? If it's the latter you're not alone. Most men aren't hot on post-sex loving. This is partly because the male sleep hormone kicks in almost immediately after ejaculation, whereas it takes 20 minutes for us women, leaving us to ponder the meaning of life on our own. If post-sex doesn't live up to pre-sex it's worth bearing in mind that long-drawn-out talks about what just happened, your latest relationship woes and/or going to dinner at your parents aren't usually success-ful at this time.

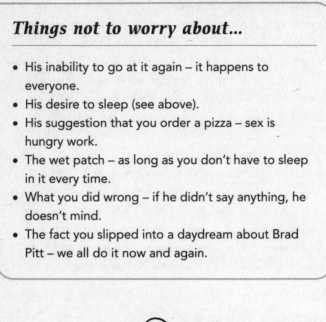

Things not to worry about...

- His inability to go at it again – it happens to everyone.
- His desire to sleep (see above).
- His suggestion that you order a pizza – sex is hungry work.
- The wet patch – as long as you don't have to sleep in it every time.
- What you did wrong – if he didn't say anything, he doesn't mind.
- The fact you slipped into a daydream about Brad Pitt – we all do it now and again.

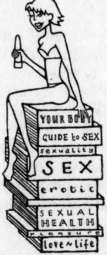

Things to worry about

1. If he falls asleep and you haven't had an orgasm yet

Selfish-lover alert. If he can't tell if you've come, or isn't bothered to check, you need to take action. Either wake him up and get him moving, or else bring up the subject the next morning. Every man likes to think he can make a woman orgasm – so shame him into at least trying. Don't whatever you do finish yourself off and not tell him.

2. Missing condoms

This means it's probably still inside you, which also means so too is his semen – cue emergency pill (see Chapter 7). Always make sure he holds the top of the condom and withdraws slowly or else the condom will slip off inside you.

3. The fact he called you someone else's name again

While slipping out the wrong name looks disastrous, the fact is it's not the end of the world, if it only happens once. If it happens more than that, and it's always the same name, either he's an idiot and can't focus on anything but his orgasm or he is fantasising about someone else. Either way tough action needs to be taken. Try pulling away, digging him in the ribs, or screaming out someone else's name (childish but it works).

facts

A study from Australia says Aussie men are choosing technology over sex. An addiction to mobiles, faxes and bleepers is said to be behind the lowering of their sex drives.

You think it's all over, but sometimes it's not

Other things you might have to worry about post-sex are:

- Post-orgasm headaches. These are very common as an orgasm causes nerve endings to fire off in the brain and muscles to tense in the neck. Ease your headaches with a cold compress to your head, or a gentle shoulder-and-neck massage from your boyfriend.
- Post-orgasm cramps. These are caused by your uterine muscles contracting as you orgasm. The more powerful your O, the bigger the cramps. These can feel similar to menstrual cramps and cause nausea. They'll pass as your body returns to its normal levels, or you could take a painkiller.
- Post-orgasm pain. If this has you doubled up it's a sign you may have a more serious condition, such as fibroids or endometriosis. See your doctor for an exact diagnosis asap.
- Post-orgasm insomnia – usually the result of very energetic sex. The no-sleep response is akin to running on a treadmill for 30 minutes and then expecting to fall asleep right away. Your body is on a cardiovascular high so you need to bring it down. Your best bet is to get up, watch TV, have a hot drink and relax until you feel sleepy.

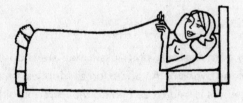

Morning-after etiquette for lazy girls

The morning after the night before is a minefield of potential disasters: shame, awkwardness and hazardous exploits all await you, especially if you don't practise the right morning etiquette.

8 ways to guarantee you'll see each other again...

1. Have a sense of humour about the night before (though obviously laugh at the right things and at the right moment).

2. Tell him you had a great time.

3. Give him a time frame for another date.

4. Be nice (even if you're Miss Grumpy in the mornings).

5. Don't freak out about the fact you had sex.

6. Don't give him a critique about his performance.

7. Be honest about what you want.

8. Go for the enjoyment factor.

8 ways to have him running for the door...

1. Talk about what you'll call your kids.

2. Go through all the things he did wrong.

3. Make fun of his bits.

4. Complain loudly about all the things wrong with your body.

5. Tell him about how you burned all your ex-boyfriend's clothes.

6. Get him to speak to your mum on the phone.

7. Ask him if you can have a photograph of him.

8. Get scary about sex.

CHAPTER SIX

The kinky stuff

WHAT'S YOUR IDEA OF KINKY SEX? Whips, chains, orgies, the erotic, the exotic, or the downright depraved? Whatever your views, the nature of kinky sex is changing big time. What used to be considered a walk on the wild side is now thought to be pretty tame. Think fluffy handcuffs on sale on the high street, TV shows featuring sex toys as the main topic of conversation, designer sleazy underwear, and body piercings galore!

While you may not be interested in whipping your boyfriend into a sexual frenzy or dressing up as a French maid, if you're like most people, you're probably more than a little curious about kinky sex and what it can do for your sex life.

While it's definitely not for everyone, adding a kinky twist is the fastest way to add a bit of zing to your sexual encounters. Thankfully this doesn't mean venturing into areas no one's ever been before (cross-dressing sex while scuba diving anyone?) but experimenting with things you've personally never done before.

The lazy girl's guide to kinky sex

According to those in the know, there is a kinky minx lurking beneath even the meekest of us, and to get to her all you have to do is act on your most creative impure and filthy thoughts. However, if you can't reach your inner kink, bear in mind it's probably only fear of being thought perverse that's holding you back.

Help Yourself By:

- Not judging yourself by other people's sexual beliefs and morals.
- Reassuring yourself that whatever you decide to try two consenting adults will be involved.
- Reasoning that being kinky about sex doesn't mean being twisted or sick about sex.
- Acknowledging you're allowed to push back your sexual boundaries.
- Admitting that sometimes you don't know what you like until you've tried it.
- Accepting that you really would like a new and different twist to your sex life.
- Reassuring yourself that risky sex doesn't mean putting yourself in danger.
- Knowing that if you don't like it, you don't have to do it again.

What being kinky can do for your sex life

1. Up your arousal levels.

2. Make you feel more confident about your sexual ability.

3. Help you feel naughty and wicked.

4. Spice up a stagnant sex life.

5. Help you find more sexual fantasies.

6. Boost your partner's desire for you.

7. Boost your desire for your partner.

8. Give you more orgasms.

9. Help you find a deeper intimacy.

10. Add some fun to your sex life.

Accessing your kinky fantasies and using them

- Read erotic fiction or porn – this can help even the least imaginative and lazy lover find scenarios to make their own. If you're too embarrassed to buy naughty fiction, look for the women-only range of books; these are graphic but aimed at females and are good for adding a little kink to your sex life.

Warning

If you are going to share fantasies, be sure to only share the ones you know your partner can handle. He doesn't need to know you fancy his best mate or dream of a threesome with your ex. Be sensitive, especially if your lover has less of a wild streak than you do. He may end up being shocked by some of your ideas.

- Let your imagination run riot. Pick a simple scenario and then just let your mind run wild. The aim is to escape from what's usual and normal for you. If you're meek and mild in bed, be dominating. See yourself in sexy clothes, dominate the sex in your dreams and imagine what it would be like to have the upper hand.
- Think about past encounters that have done it for you. The first time someone you really fancied kissed you. Try to remember the feeling, the anticipation and the outcome. Change the face of the person doing the kissing and then make him do whatever you want.
- Talk to your boyfriend about your sex dreams. If you have none of your own, use his – listen to what does it for him, and use what he's saying to turn yourself on. Try talking to him about scenarios you like (they don't have to be graphically sexual).
- Think about the Top 8 fantasies below – which ones work for you and why?

Top 8 sexual fantasies people want to make real...

1. Threesomes – usually two boys and you, if you're female. In the fantasy it's likely you get all the attention, and all the glory. The reality isn't so cut and dried – could you really handle more than one man in bed, and would it bother you if they started having sex with each other?

2. Sex with a famous person. Unless you become a groupie or take to hanging round premieres and flinging yourself at people's feet, this one's unlikely, but who cares? It's a good fantasy to use on your boyfriend (just close your eyes).

3. Sex with someone you know. Usually someone who is out of bounds – but this one could be real – so what's really holding you back? It's likely to be the fact this person's your boss/brother-in-law/best friend of your boyfriend or someone else's boyfriend/husband. If so it's best to keep this one in your head and not put it in your bed, because there's kinky sex and then there's stupid sex.

4. Sex with a stranger. Equally exciting but could be scary in reality.

5. Slave fantasies, being tied up, etc. Also sounds better in a fantasy. Though can be done if you have a very trusting partner (see page 142).

6. Same-sex sex. Lesbian encounters – a very common fantasy that does not mean you are gay even if you try it out.

7. Sex with someone watching. Also very common in fantasyland, but can you handle the reality of having your every move and body part scrutinised?

8. Sex in public. Again super common – and one that you could even make real if you're feeling brave enough, though beware of being arrested.

Pre-kinky questions

So you've talked and you've shared and now you want to act out your fantasies. Well, here's something to think about. Firstly, reality doesn't always live up to fantasy, especially if you've been replaying the same old record for the past ten years. Secondly, discuss all of the following before you give it a go.

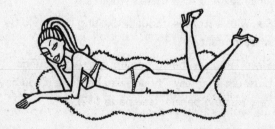

Think about what could go wrong

Spend a little time thinking about what could possibly go wrong. If you're going for a threesome, can you handle your boyfriend with someone else? What if you both enjoy it? Does this mean you're going to do it all the time?

How high are your expectations?

Talk about your expectations. Do you hope this will bring you both closer together, or are you just experimenting? Does your lover really want to do this or is he just humouring you? Does he feel under pressure to do what you want?

Is this for you?

Only you can answer this question, and the best way to do it is not to agree to do something because you're scared, frightened your boyfriend will leave, or because you know all your friends have done it. The only reason to get kinky is because you feel turned on by the thought of something.

How will you get your boyfriend to get kinky?

The worst way to get your boyfriend to take a walk on the wild side is to spring a kinky surprise on him. Men might say they like the sound of this, but suddenly brandish a whip in his direction and he's guaranteed to freak out. Instead try telling him X [add your kink] is your biggest fantasy so why don't the two of you give it a try?

What if you're not comfortable with what your boyfriend suggests?

Some things are an acquired taste, and though it may turn your stomach at first, being kinky is often a question of nothing ventured, nothing gained, so ask yourself what exactly turns you off about his request? Does it offend you? If so, say a loud 'No' because what's the point of getting turned off so he can get turned on? Does it frighten you? If so talk about it some more and get a clearer picture of what he's actually asking you to do. Maybe he's suggesting a light version and you're imagining a much darker side. However, if you are genuinely uncomfortable about doing it, don't do it, because after all, if you're not going to get turned on, what's the point?

You think being kinky is perverted and sick

Erm… you're probably best skipping this chapter.

What's what with kinky sex?

Bondage anyone?

According to the Kinsey Sex Report, over a quarter of all people are aroused by mild bondage activities. So if you've ever fantasised about being tied up, spanked, blindfolded or teased into submission you're not alone.

Mild bondage works for people because having sex with your hands bound creates anxiety and arousal in equal measure, which can only lead to a mind-blowing orgasm. Bondage also teaches even the laziest of people to be a bit more creative and the most controlling of people to let go. Best of all most men think this is pure raunchy, wicked and rampant behaviour.

"Fantasies? I just love them. They're the perfect way to wile away a boring work meeting, or drift off when you're stuck in traffic. It's amazing what your mind will come up with if you let it."

Lisa, 25

But be warned: though a bit of bondage will heighten intimacy and spice up your sex life, there are a few basics you need to be aware of before you start:

- Never tie anything that will restrict your breathing or someone else's.
- Always decide how far you are both willing to go before you start.
- Choose a word, phrase or look that you can use that will make you or your partner stop immediately if you're freaked out.
- Keep your bedroom door locked, unless you like the thrill of being caught by your flatmates.
- Never gag someone and leave him or her alone, or choke to partial asphyxiation.

How to Do it:
1. Tie or restrain your man with silk scarves or ribbons – these are better than other materials because they won't cause

friction burns on the skin. Be careful how hard you tie the binds – the aim is to fake submission, not cut off the blood supply.

2. The next step is to tease him into arousal. This means massaging and stroking his body. Move over his genital area and lick your way up and down his body and then use his body to pleasure yourself first, as this is the aim of the game.

3. Remember the whole point of doing the tying up is so you can play-act at being punishing and controlling (not take all your stress and anger out on him).

4. You have your lover at your mercy so warn him to stay silent and passive. If he speaks or moves, punish him by stopping what you're doing. He must know you're in charge of his enjoyment and ultimate satisfaction – he has to obey you, as this will heighten his orgasm potential and have him begging for more.

5. If you decide to reverse the situation, bear in mind the point of being the one tied up is that you can feign passivity and helplessness, not shout out instructions.

Good for: Control freaks who want to let go.

Role-playing

The advantages of role-playing/play-acting and dressing up can be far-reaching for your sex life. For starters it will stop boredom setting in, as it will make you both keep working at what's sexually stimulating and hot for each other. It's also a great way to reverse your usual roles. For instance, if you find that it's you who usually initiates sex then taking on a different persona could reverse this, empower your partner and add spark to your love life.

How to Do it:

1. If you want role-play to work without dissolving into a fit of laughter, you need to first work out your roles in advance because the more preparation you do the less chance you'll feel ridiculous.
2. Start by deciding who is going to be in the master role and who will be in the submissive role. Then think of a role – maybe doctor/patient, older man/younger woman, teacher/student – and work out a scenario.
3. Take it out of the bedroom. Maybe think of meeting in a bar in character, or tease each other by email all day in your roles. The more you get into the roles the more you'll get out of the sex.
4. Think about dressing up, using props, and making it as real as you can.

Good for: Creative types who need to find that extra spark.

facts

According to a new study straight out of New York, USA, while men are more likely to surf the net for porn, women are more likely to engage in cyber sex. In fact 15 per cent of women said they had tried cyber sex on more than one occasion.

Fetish delight

While fetishism conjures up images of leather-bound people in dodgy nightclubs, the truth is we all have private fixations that turn us on whether we realise it or not. Maybe you have a thing about rippling biceps, guys who wear leather pants, or men in cowboy boots (though we hope not). As bizarre as it all sounds, all a fetish is is a sexual attraction to an inanimate object or body part. A secret lust point that makes you think, 'Mmm… Yes'.

How to Do it:

1. If you have absolutely no idea what does it for your boyfriend or you, it's time for some joint experimentation. Try some joint erotic reading as a prelude to fetish fun, as these stories will show you what scenarios turn you both on. Look for elements that make you hot, such as certain clothes, underwear and parts of his body.

2. Once you've sorted out his fetish use it to your advantage, as these things will fuel his sex drive. For instance, if it's high heels and stockings that do it for him wear them when he's not expecting it. Go visit him at the office, turn up at his parents in them and tease him with the sight of them. It will become your own private sex code.

3. The only time a fetish can become a problem is if your partner can't have sex without it. Though this is rare and most people are happy just to indulge their fantasies every now and then.

Good for: Couples who want to bring sex out of the bedroom.

Voyeurism and exhibitionism

Most of us, when pushed, would admit to a
yearning for both a spot of exhibitionism
and voyeurism. This doesn't mean exposing
yourself to your neighbours or watching
them through the net curtains. It's about
taking sex, which is usually something
hidden, and making it slightly more public.

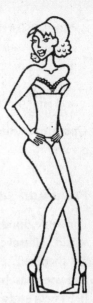

How to Do it:

1. So why not be really wicked and use a
   video camera to film your very own
   movie? Hook the camcorder up to the
   television so you can monitor the way the
   two of you look. That way you can ensure
   more flattering angles and make changes as you go
   along, rather than cringe at the result.

2. Ordinary light will do, and aim for a wide shot, so you can
   see more of the action. Once you're positioned you're free
   to do what you want and make your mark. If you feel self-
   conscious try some play-acting – talk dirty, look into the
   camera or simply make love the way you usually do. The
   aim is to see as much of each other as possible and make
   the sex look urgent and passionate.

3. If this is too brave a thought for you, try using a mirror.
   Using one during oral sex can really amplify oral sensations
   as it heightens the experience. Or place a mirror between
   his legs while you assume the top position: he can see
   himself penetrating you. The added bonus of watching
   each other is you really see what does it for him and vice
   versa.

4. Think about taking naked pictures, but avoid using a normal camera. Your local high street chemist won't be pleased if they see naked shots of you coming out of their machine. Your best bet is to use a Polaroid camera (no negatives) or a digital camera.

Good for: Attention junkies who yearn to see themselves in action.

Food and sex

For some, food and sex are the two greatest pleasures in the world. However, contrary to popular belief the two don't always mix. Use something too sharp, too sugary or too acidic and you're asking for a nasty infection down below, a possible itchy rash and a very embarrassing trip to your doctor. This is because the natural balance of the vagina is easily upset, so the more alien substances you introduce to it the more it will rebel and cause you grief. It's also worth being sensitive on the penis and nipple front. Giving your bloke a blow job while drinking champagne, very hot tea, anything with chillies or something frighteningly cold (clue: if it sticks to your hand it is too cold) will cause immediate pain,

How to Do it:

1. Phallic vegetables and fruit, like cucumbers, bananas and courgettes do make great penile substitutes. The rule is – if it's smooth and pliable and you can put a condom on it (though obviously you don't actually do this), you can use it (gently) anyway you want.

2. The key with cold food is the surprise factor – rub ice cubes on his nipples for an immediate genital hit, or suck on the

cubes, spit them out and dive south. The ice-cold sensation will literally have him gasping for more.

3. Reach for soft pulpy fruits such as strawberries, mangoes, bananas, peaches and berries. The good thing about pulpy fruit is you can smear it, eat it, lick it, grind it and massage it into the body for maximum pleasure.

4. Champagne, milkshakes, fruit juices, hot tea, and hot lemon drinks. The aim of taking a mouthful is to give your bloke a blow job while you still have a tingling sensation in your mouth and not a mouthful of liquid. Champagne and fizzy drinks can add a pain/pleasure sensation to oral sex.

Good for: Foodies.

Outdoor sex

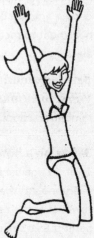

The sun's beating down on you, you're hot, you're sweaty and right now all you want to do is rip off your clothes and have sex with your bloke. And who could blame you? Sunshine boosts your levels of serotonin and testosterone – making sex all the hotter. But if you're aiming for an outdoor orgasm, it pays to pick your place carefully. Choose badly and your naked bottom could be on the front of the local newspaper.

How to Do it:

1. Sex on the beach

While water in your vagina won't do you any harm, it can literally wash away your arousal. This in turn could make sex uncomfortable and rough, so make sure you indulge in extra foreplay before you get down to it. Sex in the sea is also a far more gritty affair, and sand grains could well damage the condom prior to sex. So your best bet is to roll it on and let your bloke enter you above the surface of the water and then slide into the water together.

Best locations: Deserted beach coves and rocky beaches where you'll be partially hidden from prying eyes.
Worst locations: Beaches with loads of kids (they'll notice even if no one else will).

2. Sex in the outdoors
Try it up against something wider than your hips so no one will spot you from behind. Go for a tree with long drooping branches for maximum privacy. Having sex outside requires a certain amount of brazenness and speed – this can cause your heartbeat to race which will put your senses on hypersexual alert.

Best locations: Away from a footpath, café, car park or lake.
Worst locations: Public property – easily spotted here by ramblers, school parties and park wardens.

3. Sex on a hotel balcony
Try it up against the railings, at night, or during the day when everyone's at the beach. If your railings are sparse, drape a towel over the balcony to shield you from nosy neighbours. Semi-public sex creates anxiety and sexual tension in equal measures, which in turn boosts arousal levels and blood flow to the genitals. However, note that the chances of being seen by your neighbours or from the street are high.

Best locations: A balcony on the top floor that overlooks a beach view.

Worst locations: A balcony that overlooks the pool, the bar or another hotel.

Good for: Adding spice to your sex life.

Sex toys

Venture into any sex shop and you'll see a whole host of sex toys there for your supposed enjoyment. Vibrators, dildos, fake vaginas, fake breasts and even strange ball-shaped objects. En masse they are likely to turn you off rather than turn you on, because let's face it they look more than a little odd. However, sex toys are now a mass-market item – there are so many of them simply because so many people buy them. If they take your fancy, you have nothing to feel ashamed or guilty about. Sex toys are not a sign that you're depraved, desperate or sex starved, they are just an extension of sex. Their purpose is to enhance your sex life not replace it or be a long-term substitute for it.

How to Do it:

1. First get your sex toys right: a vibrator is a phallic-shaped device that vibrates and massages the body. A dildo is a penis-shaped version of an erect penis. Ben Wa balls are small balls that are said to give a woman sexual pleasure when inserted into the vagina. A cock ring is a rubber band that is put on the base of the penis to keep it erect for longer, and a butt plug is basically what the name says.

2. If you fancy your chances with one of the above and can't bear shopping on the high street for one, you can easily buy them from mail-order catalogues and the Internet, and

have them delivered in a nondescript brown package (see Resources).

3. The benefit of sex toys is they can help you reach greater sexual bliss as they can help you find your sexually sensitive areas and aid arousal, so don't just keep them for private but introduce them into your sex life. Though don't share them, as this is a good way to spread bacteria and infection.

Good for: Those looking for that elusive orgasm.

facts

In Arizona, USA, the law states you cannot have more than two vibrators in one house.

Talking dirty

This is not about letting off a stream of expletives and generally being crude and rude about sex (unless this is what does it for you). It's a way of using language to incite sexual arousal. This means thinking up sexually enticing words and lewd scenarios, and generally working your way down to the more expressive phrases. It works so well because it conjures up instant verbal pictures, creates sexual tension and can be used wherever you are via text messages, emails (though be wary if you're using a work email program) and the phone.

How to Do it:

1. The most important thing about talking dirty is to first find out what you and your boyfriend find acceptable. After all

it's no good both of you trying to outdo each other if one of you ends up offended and turned off.

2. Stuck for what to say? Then read some erotica, and think about what would turn you on. Or take it at it's easiest form: call him at work and start off by telling your boyfriend what you're going to do to him when you get him home, recount past scenarios, embellish your story and generally make him hot just by the sound of your voice.

3. Can't say the words? Then think about making more appreciative sounds during sex. Moans and groans are super effective at getting your pleasure across.

Good for: Long-distance lovers and those who want to make sex an all-day experience.

Dirty movies, also known as pornography

Pornography is one of the grey areas of sex. While around 50 per cent of couples happily use it, lots of people find it deeply offensive, sexist and abusive. Whatever your take, if you don't like it, don't feel you have to watch it or use it. Pornography, like everything else to do with sex, is a choice.

How to Use it:

1. Firstly work out what type of film you want to watch. Soft porn is basically the stuff you see on TV and at the movies. Then you have your mid-porn which is basically your standard sex film with dodgy story lines about couples having sex with a few lesbian and group sex encounters thrown in. Finally you have what's known as hardcore – the movies that many people (even those who use pornography) find offensive because they are 100 per cent graphic and do reach the borders of depravity.

2. Bear in mind all porn films get pretty dull after a while because there are no plots, the dialogue stinks and of course the acting is limited. This is because the whole point is the sex. The aim is to watch, get turned on, get some ideas and have sex.

3. If films don't do it for you, think about magazines. Many women don't like these and hate their boyfriends using them. If this is the case with your relationship, it's worth bearing in mind that the magazines are for visual stimuli and not because your boyfriend would rather be dating one of the surgically enhanced women inside.

Good for: Couples stuck for sex ideas.

facts

The online sex industry generates one billion US dollars a year.

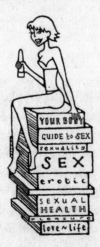

A lazy girl's guide to kinky sexual dilemmas

1. Is it polite to bring a vibrator to bed?

When it comes to bedmates of the mechanical kind, most men consider two's company, and three's a crowd. However, if you're still tempted, remember: though vibrators work as an antidote to crap sex, even the dimmest of lovers will notice a loud buzzing noise coming from your side of the bed.

2. Is it okay to finish off the job with a sex toy if he hasn't done it for me?

Most definitely, but only if you make it a performance. This will not only give him some much-needed pointers in the how-to-make-my-girlfriend-happy department, but it will also make him think you're doing all this just for his benefit.

3. Is it offensive to laugh when he talks dirty?

Even the most wanton of lovers will become unresponsive fast if you make fun of their sexual turn-ons. Not convinced? Then ask yourself this: is it offensive for him to laugh when you come out in sexy underwear?

4. How dirty can you get in bed before offending your boyfriend?

If you've already reached the borders of depravity and it's your second date, then it's likely nothing will be too much. However, if he insists on having sex on a towel and with the lights off, then resist anything more adventurous than the missionary position.

5. My boyfriend keeps suggesting we have sex somewhere dangerous and unconventional. Should I let him choose the location?

If you trust him with simple things, like choosing your holidays, then you're probably safe. Though be sure to remind him that the fun lies in the risk of getting caught, not in risking one's life! If not, take control of the situation immediately, otherwise you could find yourself having sex under a CCTV camera.

6. My boyfriend is always suggesting we go for it in the bathroom when we're at his parent's house or trying to have sex under the table at restaurants. What is this about?

It sounds like your boyfriend has started to associate hot sex with danger. What you need to do is find out which part of public sex turns him on the most. Is it the naughty boy element, the being watched aspect or the fact he can potentially entice you into sex anywhere he wants? Once you've worked this out, you can use this at home. If he likes the fact you may be seen by others, turn the lights off and open your curtains as you have sex – this will give you a similar feeling to being in the open, without literally being in the open.

7. My boyfriend keeps suggesting a threesome with one of my friends. When I say I don't think so he says I'm a sexual prude.

Suggest a threesome with one of his mates and see how he responds. While two girls in a bed is the number-one male fantasy, the chances are he'll more than see your point if you turn the tables on him. If he doesn't, be wary: group sex is just around the corner!

8. I sometimes want to punish my boyfriend – is this a sexual thing?

It depends on why and when you want to punish your boyfriend. If you feel like beating him every time he flirts with other women then this is unlikely to be a sexual urge. However, if you like the idea of being in control in bed and punishing him in a fake scenario then you're talking sex.

9. How kinky can you get?

As kinky as a consenting partner allows you to be. However, it's worth noting while getting comfy about sex is the kiss of death to a relationship, breaking the law in order to get your sexual kicks (even if you consider your behaviour to be harmless) will get you arrested.

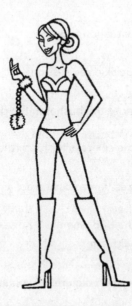

25 ways
to get kinky without trying to hard

1. Dress up.

2. Dress down.

3. Talk dirty.

4. Pay him a surprise visit at work during his lunch hour.

5. Role-play a situation together.

6. Instigate a quickie sex session.

7. Drag him under the bushes in the park.

8. Buy him some sex toys for his birthday.

9. Access his best fantasies and act it out for him.

10. Tie him to the bed when he's not expecting it and start having sex with him.

11. Drop some naked pictures of yourself into his lap.

12. Buy some sexy his-and-her underwear.

13. Bring a friend to bed (if you dare).

14. Suggest you make a home movie together.

15. Write him a filthy love letter and leave it in his diary or bag.

16. Drag him into the bedroom for a session at your parents' house.

17. Tell him you're not wearing knickers today.

18. Indulge in some phone sex together.

19. Experiment with a vibrator.

20. Buy some handcuffs and leave them hanging from the bed.

21. Bring some whipped cream and ice cream to bed.

22. Ask him what he's thinking as you get undressed.

23. Tell him what you're thinking as you get undressed.

24. Go on a sex-starvation diet where all you can do is talk about it all week.

25. Spend a whole weekend in bed together – you'll be amazed at where it will take you both.

CHAPTER SEVEN

The sensible stuff

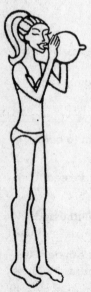

CONTRACEPTION IS ALL ABOUT CHOICES. Not the choice of whether to go bareback or not, but the choice of what to use, what not to use and whether or not to protect yourself from sexual nasties (STIs). Even the laziest among us knows we should use contraception, but finding the ideal method can be a drag. Maybe you hate the thought of condoms or are worried that the pill makes you fat. Perhaps IUDs leave you cold or the cap seems like too much of an effort to use. Whatever your worry, the good news is contraception is becoming easier to get and safer to use, all thanks to new scientific advances, better designs and changes in the hormonal mixes of methods such as the pill. This means even if you're someone who thinks nothing works for them, the truth is something will – all you have to do is give it a try.

Why you should use contraception

- It's easier than dealing with a cauliflower growth on your genitals.
- It's free and easy to get hold of.
- It's easier than having a baby.
- It will protect the sexual health of the person you love as well as yours.
- It will stop any embarrassing trips to your GP.
- It will help you avoid bad smells and discharges down below.
- It will keep you fertile.
- It will keep sex pain-free.
- It will stop you infecting future lovers.
- It will stop you passing on diseases to your baby when you're ready to have one.
- It will protect you from cervical cancer.

What's not contraception?

First a quick word about what's not contraception. No matter how old you are, myths abound about what works and what doesn't when it comes to contraception. The largest area of dissent seems to be around the matter of withdrawal. This is where a guy withdraws his penis before ejaculating thereby aiming to leave no sperm inside you. The problem with this is simply that pre-ejaculatory semen also contains sperm, plus you have to have a boyfriend who absolutely knows what he's doing – otherwise he'll withdraw too late. Plus – and this is a biggie – withdrawal offers no protection against sexually transmitted diseases. So if you're with a guy who's adept at withdrawing it means he practises withdrawal a lot, and so has had unprotected sex a lot – and we all know what that means!

And what is?

The pill

This is basically a hormonal method of contraception. It contains two hormones – oestrogen and progestogen – which prevent an egg from being released by a woman's ovary each month. It is highly effective when used properly but offers no protection against STIs and HIV.

It's estimated that 70 million women worldwide take the pill, because it's the most foolproof method of contraception available.

The pill facts

1. The pill is more likely to benefit your general health than damage it

In fact, it will not only improve your skin, reduce period cramping and heavy blood loss, but it will also help you to stay fertile longer. One recent study has even suggested women who take the pill for more than nine years before the age of thirty may have a significant decrease in the risk of miscarriage when they do become pregnant.

facts

Percentage of women using contraception:

Australia 72

New Zealand 72

South Africa 48

UK 82

US 67

France 69

Spain 38

2. It's safe

So why all the fuss? In October 1995, the Committee on Safety of Medicines reported that the relative risk of developing the life-threatening venous thromboembolism was twice as high among women taking the pill. However, to put this scare in perspective, normal pregnancy increases the risk of thromboembolism twice as much as the pill. The actual risk of dying from pill use is between one in half a million and one in a million. This is equivalent to the chance of being killed in a train crash, or being struck by lightning, and ten times less likely than being murdered.

3. What about side effects?

It's also worth knowing that today's pills are safer than ever: they have much lower dosages of hormones, and some even carry only one type of hormone; all of which helps combat the various side effects, such as nausea and headaches, which are often associated with taking the pill.

"I'm on the pill and just knowing that if I take it properly I won't get pregnant has really improved my sex life."

Kim, 28

How the pill works

Combined pills contain the hormones, oestrogen and progesterone and when taken stop ovulation. This means the pill tricks your body into thinking you are pregnant, so your own hormones aren't released to start up your menstrual cycle. Alongside this, the pill activates the build-up of cervical mucus so sperm cannot get through, and a fertilised egg (if there is one) cannot implant itself in the womb lining.

Most pill packs are designed to last a month and every pill contains exactly the same amount of hormone. This means you take one pill every day for three weeks and then you take a week off (in some brands you have to take placebo pills during this week). During this week off, the womb lining will be expelled and you get a period, though not a real period because ovulation has not occurred.

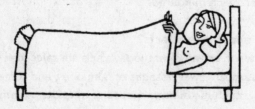

The pill — health bonuses

- Regular periods.
- Less bleeding.
- Less or no cramping.
- Clearer skin.
- Lower incidence of breast cancer, ovarian cancer and endometrial cancer.
- Lower risk of pelvic inflammatory disease.
- Fewer ovarian cysts.
- May help to preserve fertility.
- Builds stronger bones.
- Reduces heavy bleeding from periods.
- Reduces iron deficiency anaemia.
- Stops you from getting pregnant.

Pill myths

Myth: *It makes you put on weight*
Studies show women are just as likely to lose weight as gain weight while on the pill. Weight gain, if there is any, usually only occurs in the first month as your body adjusts to the contraceptive. If weight gain continues, it's likely you need to be on a different pill, with a different hormonal dosage.

Myth: *It's bad for you to go directly from one pack to the next, without taking a week off for a period*
Strangely enough there is nothing necessary about this period. In the early days, the pill was developed to copy the menstrual cycle because manufacturers believed most women

would still want to take a pill that allowed them to mimic the natural 28-day cycle. This means you can safely take the pill without a monthly bleed, though you should always check with your GP first.

Myth: *The pill gives you lots of side effects, like nausea and headaches*
Some pills can give you side effects (but bear in mind all drugs and medicines can give you side effects), but lots of women have none. If you're suffering, see your doctor in order to change to a pill with a different hormonal dosage.

Myth: *Taking more than one will give you double protection*
Taking a double dose will not give you double protection. However, if you forget to take a pill (and 47 per cent of women do) you can take it as long as it's not more than 12 hours late. For delays longer than this, always check with your GP. It is 99 per cent effective if used correctly.

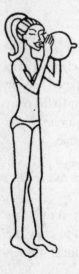

Condoms

Made of very thin latex rubber, condoms work by being placed over the penis. They act as a physical barrier and trap sperm at the point of ejaculation. They help to protect against cancer of the cervix and reduce the risk of STIs, including HIV.

New condoms

Love using condoms but hate the smell? Well you're not alone – so, thank goodness, some boffin has come up with the ideal solution: an odour mask to eliminate that pungent smell of rubber. Better still, look out for the 'Ez-ON', a new roomy American condom that is already available in Holland. This condom has a wider fitting and doesn't roll on but is pulled on like a sock. Pros include the fact it offers greater vaginal stimulation, and a potential G-spot hit.

Try a polyurethane condom. These are new condoms that are made from the same material as the female condom – Femidom. They are thinner and stronger.

Condom facts

- The condom will protect you from STIs, pregnancy and HIV.
- Only ever use water-based lubricants, such as KY jelly, with condoms.
- Vaseline, body oils and lotions can erode latex, making it tear more easily.
- Always store condoms in a cool place; heat also erodes latex.

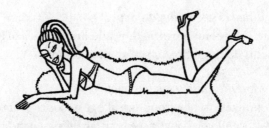

How to use a condom

1. Do not roll on a condom until he is erect (also do not unravel one and attempt to place it over the penis).
2. Squeeze the tip to get rid of the air, place on head of penis and gently roll down over the penis to the base, smoothing out bubbles as you go (air bubbles can cause the condom to break).
3. Ensure your partner withdraws as soon as possible after ejaculation, holding the condom in place at the base, so it doesn't slip off.
4. Never reuse a condom.
5. If a condom splits, tears or slips off inside you always make sure you take precautions and use the emergency pill.
6. Only use condoms approved with the UK BSI kite mark symbol or the symbol of approval for your country, as these show they have been tested to national minimum standards of quality.

Condom myths

Myth: *It makes sex uncomfortable*
Not true – condoms are ultra thin, and once stretched over an erect penis does not hinder sex or ejaculation.

Myth: *Most men find them too tight*
Highly unlikely – blow one up like a balloon if you don't believe me, and you'll really see how far they stretch.

facts

A study from the University of Sydney, Australia, found that men were more likely to break condoms if:

(1) they didn't use them very often, and

(2) pulled the condom on, rather than rolling it on.

Myth: *They don't work anyway*
Totally untrue – use them properly (see instructions on page 168) and they work very effectively. If used according to instructions, condoms are 98 per cent effective.

The female condom

Known as the Femidom, the female condom is a tube-like structure with two rings either end. The small end fits into the vagina and the big end hangs outside of the vagina, so that the whole of the vagina is protected. Some people complain it's like having sex inside a bag, but the truth is the female condom is made of very thin polyurethane (not latex), and as long as you hold it in place as your boyfriend enters he will not slip under it and it won't slip when he withdraws. The female condom is 98 per cent effective when used correctly.

Diaphragm/cap

The diaphragm is a circular dome made of rubber that is used with spermicidal cream and fitted over the cervix to stop sperm from getting into the uterus. You can put it in any time before sex, but a trained nurse must initially fit it. Fitting should be checked every year, and/or if you gain or lose more than 3kg (7lb) or have a baby. It is 96 per cent effective when used correctly.

IUD (intrauterine device)

This small plastic and copper device, usually shaped like a T or 7, works from the moment it is placed in the uterus and can stay in place for five years. The only problem is some IUDs may cause periods to be heavier, and sometimes the IUD can be expelled by the womb. If this occurs you will be at risk of pregnancy as soon as you have sex. IUDs are 98–99 per cent effective.

For those who have had a bad experience with intrauterine devices (IUDs), GyneFIX is a new type of IUD. It has a short row of copper beads, which bend to fit the inside of the uterus instead of being T-shaped like most IUDs. Once properly inserted, it causes less painful side effects than traditional IUDs and can be used either as a long-term contraceptive, staying in place for five years, or as an emergency method of contraception within five days of unprotected intercourse.

IUS (intrauterine system)

This is a small plastic device, which contains the hormone progestogen. It is effective as soon as it is placed in the womb and lasts for at least three years. Very useful for women with painful, heavy periods as it makes periods lighter, but sporadic bleeding is common for the first three months. There may be temporary side effects, like acne and breast tenderness. It is 99 per cent effective.

Implant

An implant is a small soft tube, the size of a matchstick, which is placed under the skin of the upper arm. It then releases a steady flow of the hormone progestogen into the blood-stream.

You are protected from pregnancy for up to five years. Implants are unsuitable for women who are at risk from stroke, heart disease, liver disease or breast or ovarian cancer. They are 99 per cent effective in the first year of use, 98 per cent effective over five years.

Contraceptive injection

This is an injection of hormones that provides a longer-acting alternative to the pill. It works by slowly releasing the hor-mone progestogen into the body to stop ovulation. It is injected into a muscle, usually in your bottom.

You don't have to think about contraception for as long as the injection lasts, but possible side effects include weight gain and irregular bleeding. It is 99 per cent effective.

Natural methods

(The rhythm method, the basal body temperature method, the Billings/cervical mucus method.)

This is where you count your fertile and unfertile days. Once you have that information you must then avoid sex (or use a method of contraception) on fertile days. There are no harmful side effects and it can be used at any stage of a woman's reproductive life, as long as your menstrual cycle is regular. Only suitable for women who are very organised and have regular periods, otherwise it has a high failure rate. Natural methods are 98 per cent effective if used according to instructions.

"I have a friend who tried the natural method of contraception and got pregnant – I'm certainly not going to risk it because I can't be bothered to work out my ovulation patterns properly."

Louise, 26

Emergency contraception

There are two methods of preventing pregnancy after unprotected sex and both have to be started within one to five days – though the sooner you sort it out the more effective the contraceptive will be.

The emergency pill

Available from your local chemist, your GP and family planning clinics.

If unprotected sex occurs within 72 hours (three days), get the emergency contraceptive pill. The newest pill, Levonelle-2, has only two pills, unlike the old emergency pill, PC4, which contained four pills.

The benefits of this pill are:

- It doesn't make you feel sick or cause you to throw up.
- It's also 95 per cent effective and holds no health risks. This pill stops conception happening (it won't work if you are already pregnant) and is not the same as the abortion pill, which is not available over the counter.

IUD

If you've waited beyond 72 hours but under five days, an IUD can be inserted by a doctor into the uterus to prevent the lining of the womb from thickening. This will halt conception. This is an effective post-sex method and its contraceptive value can last three years (or you can have it removed again).

What's new in contraception?

The contraceptive patch

Evra is a patch very like the nicotine patch and is preferably worn on your bottom or your arm. It delivers a continuous flow of the hormones oestrogen and progestogen directly through your skin into your bloodstream.

All you have to do is wear it for seven days at a time and then take a break every three weeks. The main disadvantage is the fact that Evra offers no protection from STIs.

The vaginal ring

NuvaRing is a hollow, flexible ring with a very thin circumference filled with hormones and designed to fit near your cervix. Advantages of the ring include the fact it delivers the hormones direct to the right spot (i.e. the cervix and uterus), meaning all those hormones don't travel through the body giving you nasty side effects like breast tenderness and mood swings. Disadvantages: no STI protection.

Smart hormones

Currently being researched, these hormones are smart by name and smart by nature. It's hoped they will work directly on the exact reproductive cell and organ in your body without affecting surrounding cells and organs. You rub them into the skin and they home in to your reproductive organs; meaning no side effects, lower doses and near-perfect contraception.

Vaginal microbicides

Microbicides are the space-age arm of contraception and will one day work by killing off all sexual infections and sperm. They are likely to be administered via a pessary and though they are still some way off, a version is currently on trial in South Africa (though not for contraceptive purposes but to see if it can fight off the HIV infection).

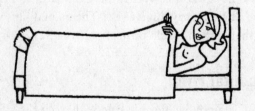

Scratch that itch — sexually transmitted infections explained

They're on the rise, they're highly contagious and they cause everything from embarrassing itches to fertility problems. Here's why safer sex is a girl's best friend.

Sexual infection checklist

- Make sure you and a new partner are checked out and cleared of infection before you start having unprotected sex.
- If an STI is present, avoid sex until you have both been treated for the infection and you have both been given the all clear.
- Always use a barrier method of contraception if you have sex with someone you don't know is clear.
- Don't assume you're clear just because you have no symptoms.
- Don't play Russian roulette with your sex life — have unprotected sex with enough people and you'll soon catch something nasty.
- Be aware that sexual infections don't always present symptoms. Signs to watch out for are:
  - mysterious genital lumps and bumps.
  - vaginal blisters — small or large.
  - discharges — watery or lumpy or smelly.
  - irritation — anywhere in the genital region.
  - strange smells — especially if it's fishy.
  - rashes around the genital area (not just the vagina, but the bottom and upper thighs).

- pain during sex – contrary to popular belief this is not normal.
- lumps, rashes and discharges from the penis.
- painful urination.
- Visit your nearest GUM (genito-urinary medicine) clinic for help. GUM clinics are 100 per cent confidential. Though they are usually situated in a hospital, the records held there never leave the clinic. This means they are not placed with your normal hospital records or sent to your GP. So no one will ever known you've been.
- If you're ever unsure about something, get it checked out. Sexual infections (both STIs and genito-urinary infections) are easily treated but spread quickly so the sooner they are caught and dealt with the better.

Sexually transmitted infections

STIs, unlike genito-urinary infections (see pages 180–83), are passed only through sex and genital contact. The problem with STIs is they often present no symptoms and though most can be treated with antibiotics and anti-virals, some, such as HIV, genital warts and genital herpes, cannot be cured, though they can be controlled with medication.

Chlamydia

The latest figures show that cases of chlamydia have soared in recent years. If you've never heard of it you're not alone. Some studies estimate that 5 per cent of all sexually active young people are infected with this STI and don't know it. This means there could be around 150,000 young women in the

UK alone with chlamydia; a scary thought because, if left untreated, chlamydia can lead to pelvic inflammatory disease and infertility.

The infection begins on the cervix and, unless it is diagnosed and treated, it spreads to the Fallopian tubes (the tubes along which an egg passes to get to the womb) and results in pelvic inflammatory disease (PID). It is PID that then leads to problems with fertility, as the Fallopian tubes become blocked and scarred as a result of the disease. Once this occurs, fertilised eggs cannot reach the uterus and you cannot get pregnant.

Chlamydia, though highly infectious and dangerous, can be diagnosed with a simple test and treated effectively with just one course of antibiotic tablets.

Symptoms: Possible symptoms to look out for (though these occur in only 20 per cent of cases):

- Breakthrough bleeding between the menstrual cycle.
- Vaginal bleeding after sex.
- Abdominal pain.
- Low-grade fever.
- Abnormal discharge.
- Pain when you urinate.
- Men may find a small, milky discharge and burning while urinating.

Genital warts

This type of wart is a particularly virulent STI. The small fleshy growths can appear anywhere on the genital area and are caused by a virus called human papilloma virus (HPV).

Symptoms: Warts usually take between one and three months to appear. If you have them, you might notice small, white lumps or a cauliflower-shaped lump. They may itch but are usually painless.

The big problem with warts is there are often no symptoms, or the warts develop inside the vagina (usually on the cervix) so you can't see them, and then they can lead to all sorts of problems (see cervical cancer below).

Diagnosis: A doctor/nurse can usually tell if you have warts through an internal examination. However, because warts are viral, antibiotics will not get rid of them. Treatment is usually through freezing or laser treatment.

facts

A new law that insists you wear condoms has come into effect in Bavaria. As prostitution is legal in Germany, the health minister has passed a law saying all men must wear condoms to prevent the spread of disease.

Herpes

The herpes simplex virus (HSV) causes genital herpes. There is no cure for herpes and the virus can affect the mouth, the genital area and the anus. There are two types of this virus: type I, which usually causes cold sores, and type II that causes genital sores. Kissing passes herpes type I. Herpes type II is passed through sex. Though type I becomes type II through oral sex.

Symptoms: Small blisters on the genital region, which eventually become sores, pain when passing urine, flu-like illness and headaches.

Diagnosis: A sample is taken and you may be given a pelvic examination. Tablets will then be given to reduce the HSV infection. Remember, HSV is highly infectious and during an outbreak you should avoid sex and kissing (if you have cold sores).

Gonorrhoea

This disease affects both men and women, and in five out of every six cases there are no symptoms. The danger of this is that it can cause pelvic inflammatory disease if left undiagnosed.

Symptoms: A vaginal or penile discharge and a burning sensation when passing urine. Sore genital region; sometimes a sore throat.

Diagnosis: Samples are usually taken from the genital region. If you have gonorrhoea you will be given penicillin to treat it.

HIV and AIDS

According to a new MORI poll 51 per cent of UK women do not think of using a condom before starting a new sexual relationship. Not wise, considering the latest statistics show HIV infection figures are on the increase, especially among young heterosexual people.

Help yourself: By practising safer sex and limiting your sexual partners.

Trichomoniasis

This is a sexually transmitted infection, which needs anti-bacterial drugs in order to be cleared up.

Symptoms: Characterised by a vile-smelling yellow-green discharge, trichomoniasis has symptoms similar to thrush, with itching and a thick discharge.

Genito-urinary infections

Infections that are not sexually transmitted but can be passed on through sex are known as genito-urinary infections. These include cystitis, bladder infections, vaginal thrush and bacterial vaginosis.

Symptoms: The main symptoms of cystitis are burning and stinging when you pass urine, for thrush a white, curdy discharge and for bacterial vaginosis a greyish-white discharge with a fishy smell. All can be treated easily with antibiotics and antifungal medication.

While many of these can be treated over the counter it's wise not to self-diagnose. It's easy to assume a discharge is something you know, such as thrush, but beware: a discharge could be one of the most common sexually transmitted vaginal infections – trichomoniasis. If you suspect you may be infected with anything, go to your nearest GUM clinic for a diagnosis.

Bacterial vaginosis

Also known as gardnerella, bacterial vaginosis is a very common bacterial infection that arises spontaneously within the body when a normal type of bacteria overgrows in the vagina. Certain things help this to happen including, douching, bubble baths and having the coil fitted.

Symptoms: A bad-smelling fishy discharge with a watery yellow to greyish tint. Some women say it's worse after a period and having sex, and in some cases there is itching around the vulva. It's estimated that 5–30 per cent of women carry BV with no symptoms, which means, this amount of women could have a possible flare-up.

Treatment is easy: Go to your doctor's or your local GUM clinic (genito-urinary medicine clinic, found at your local hospital) and the infection will be treated with an antibiotic or with a vaginal cream.

Cystitis

This is an inflammation of the bladder, which is why sufferers always experience a frequent and painful urge to pee. It's caused by bacteria, which usually live in the bowel and anus, spreading to the urethra and bladder.

While very common and irritating, cystitis isn't going to damage your sexual health, though it can be recurring, so prevention is always the best way of dealing with it.

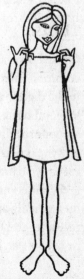

Avoid cystitis by:

- Going to the bathroom for a pee both before and immediately after sex. This helps flush away the bacteria that cause cystitis.

- If you're prone to attacks, avoid rough sex, or sex which involves a lot of thrusting, as this can cause small tears near the urethra and allow infection to get in and spread.
- Always make sure you're well lubricated, as lubrication will also help avoid the above.
- Make sure your boyfriend hasn't got urethritis – the male version of cystitis. Symptoms include pain on peeing and ejaculation.

If you do get cystitis don't immediately just go for the over-the-counter medication. If it lasts more than 48 hours, see your doctor for antibiotics, because some bouts need stronger medication.

- During an outbreak drink plenty of water – a glass every half an hour, as it's essential you flush out the bladder.
- Drink cranberry juice, which is a urinary antiseptic.

Thrush

Caused by a fungus called candida albicans, thrush is a common infection. Usually this fungus lives quite harmlessly in the digestive tract of most people and is kept under control by good bacteria in the gut. The problem with candida is it's an opportunistic infection, which means it takes advantage of any weakness or imbalance in the body. Symptoms are extreme itchiness and a thick cottage-cheese-like discharge (very different from a normal vaginal discharge). Thrush in men usually appears as an itch around the head of the penis or under the foreskin. More severe symptoms might be red, dry, flaky patches and/or a swelling on the head of the penis.

How you can get rid of it: Once you have been diagnosed with thrush, you can buy an over-the-counter cream or pessary, such as Canesten (Clotrimazole) or Diflucan (Fluconazole). With antifungal treatment like this, thrush can be eliminated within a week. The success rate for these antifungal treatments is over 90 per cent, so if one cream doesn't work, you should try another.

Some women gain short-term relief by applying natural yoghurt to the genital area. This works, as it calms the area down, but there is no scientific proof that it will get rid of thrush and, therefore, yoghurt is no substitute for antifungal medication.

How to prevent thrush

By far the best way to deal with thrush is prevention:

- Wear natural fibres, such as cotton, next to the genital area and avoid very tight trousers and tights, as these give the fungus warm conditions for growth.
- Avoid heavily perfumed soaps and bubble baths as these can irritate the vaginal area. This also means not washing your hair in the bath.
- If your thrush is recurring, always see your GP for further tests and advice.

Escape general vaginal infections by saying no to...

Douching

This is a method whereby you squirt water or other supposed 'helpful' fluid into the vagina in order to cleanse it. It's a totally useless and quite harmful thing to do for three reasons: (1) as long as you're hygienic and wash regularly there's no need to worry about cleansing the vagina, (2) any liquid entering the vagina is more likely to muck up the natural pH balance of the vagina and cause an infection like thrush, and (3) if you do have a bacterium lurking in your pants, all douching will do is help it on its way round your vagina.

The wrong type of lubricant

Okay, you probably know the spiel – Vaseline, body lotion and bath oil are all no-nos for sexual lubricants as they eat away at condoms. But they are also a bad idea to use during sex because they can cause a very nasty itch down below. Perfumed products in particular can also cause thrush and an allergic response in the vagina. Remember the genital area is about as delicate as your face and should be treated as such.

Rough sex

It may be hot sex to you, but rough sex can also cause some microscopic tears around the genital area, which act as access points for bacterial infections. The tears near the urethra are particularly troublesome as they allow bacteria into the bladder and this is how cystitis occurs. Help yourself by always using a condom if you're attempting something primal and wild, and by peeing before and after sex, to help cast out any nasties that may have worked their way into your bladder.

Vaginal deodorants

The vagina has a natural musky smell and isn't meant to smell of roses. Deodorants may mask smells but they also upset the delicate pH balance of the vagina and irritate the vaginal tissues.

Essential sexual health checks

Keep young and beautiful by ensuring your insides stay as fresh and healthy as your outsides. If, like the majority of the female population, you'd choose to stick your head down the toilet before having a smear test/breast test or even pelvic examination, you should think again. These tests can literally save your life.

HPV genital warts test

The principal culprit of cervical cancer is thought to be the human papilloma virus (HPV), otherwise known as genital warts (implicated in up to 93 per cent of cervical cancer cases). There is now a test, which is 95 per cent accurate in detecting HPV. It is thought that by doing this at the same time as a smear, cervical cancer could one day be eradicated.

Breast examination

Cancer of the breast affects 1 in 12 women, which is why it's essential to check your breasts regularly in the following way:

1. Moving in a circular motion, cover the whole breast area from deep in the armpit over the top of the breast tissue.
2. Remember to move centrally and underneath the breast, finally circling around and over the nipple.
3. It is also important to feel around the collarbone and into the armpit for any swellings.
4. Look for:
   - Appearance changes in your breast such as puckering and dimpling.
   - Feelings of breast discomfort.
   - Lumps.
   - Nipple discharge and change in the nipple position.
   - A breast lump. Unlike cysts, which tend to be firm, well defined and tender, breast lumps are usually hard and painless.
   - Don't expect the lumps to be large; in 51 per cent of cases, lumps were less than 3cm (1.25in) in size.

Chlamydia test

The most common sexually transmitted infection among women is chlamydia. It's now estimated that 5 per cent of all sexually active people are infected but don't realise it because there are rarely any symptoms. If left untreated chlamydia can lead to pelvic inflammatory disease (PID) and infertility. The test (usually involving a swab or urine sample) is quick, and the infection is treated effectively with just one course of antibiotic tablets.

Pelvic examination

This is a routine diagnostic check of the health of your pelvic region performed by a doctor both manually (with two fingers) and with a speculum. This test should be done regularly after the age of 35, especially if you have one of the following: pelvic pain, bladder problems, irregular bleeding, unusual discharge, pain during sex and/or suspect you may have an STI.

Cervical smears

This test is basically an internal examination whereby a nurse/doctor takes cells from the cervix in order to test for any possible changes, which could indicate pre-cancerous cells. If changes can be detected at an early stage, cancer can then be avoided altogether. As scary as this sounds, the good news is that, according to the latest figures, 91.4 per cent of women tested in the UK are given the all-clear right away.

Is it painful? Smears are more uncomfortable than painful, mainly because of a device called a speculum, which is inserted into your vagina. This instrument, though torturous-looking is used simply to separate the walls of the vagina so a doctor/nurse can see the condition of your cervix. A wooden spatula is then wiped across the cervix (neck of the womb) to scrape off cells. These cells are then smeared onto a glass slide and sent to a laboratory to be examined.

What happens after the test? A few weeks after a smear test, your results will be sent to you. The results are likely to note one of five things:

1. Inadequate – which means the nurse/doctor did not manage to pick up enough cells to get a proper report. If this happens, there is nothing to worry about and all you have to do is go back for another test.
2. Negative – this gives you the all-clear, and you don't have to have another test for three to five years.
3. Mild dysplasia or borderline reading – this means an infection may be present and you should be screened more regularly, usually every six months.
4. Moderate dysplasia – this shows inflammation in the cells and a need for more investigation.
5. Severe dysplasia – means there are detectable changes in the cells and you need some treatment.

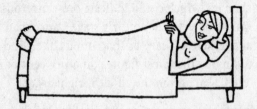

6 ways to make going for a cervical smear test easier

1. Wear a skirt. Sounds obvious, but this is a quicker and slightly less embarrassing way to make sure you're in and out of the surgery quickly.
2. Make an appointment with a female doctor or nurse. Even if your doctor is a man you do not have to see him for your smear and can opt for a female doctor/nurse.
3. Ask the doctor/nurse to warm the speculum before it's inserted. This makes the insertion less of a shock to the system.
4. Drop your tailbone and try to relax. Due to nerves, many women tense before the speculum is inserted, making it more uncomfortable and difficult to adjust. One way to make insertion easier is to concentrate on dropping your tailbone (imagine the base of your spine and your bottom resting flat on the bed).
5. Speak up if it's painful. Again it sounds obvious, but speak up if it hurts because the doctor may need to use a smaller speculum.
6. Avoid sex the night before you go. This is because semen makes the smear results unreliable (as does blood so avoid going when you have a period).

What causes cervical cancer? There are a number of possible factors that have been linked to cervical cancer, including sex and smoking. However, the principal culprit is thought to be the human papilloma virus (HPV), otherwise known as genital warts. Several types of HPV have been found to cause cervical cancer, and these have been implicated in up to 93 per cent of cervical cancer cases. Other risk factors for cervical cancer include smoking, because carcinogens – cancer-causing chemicals absorbed from cigarette smoke – are excreted in fluid produced by the cervix. It's this inter-action that can lead the cells of the cervix to change.

Cervical Cancer Vaccine

From 2008, girls in year 8 at school (aged 12 to 13 years) will be offered the new HPV vaccine in the UK, known as Cervarix. Girls will have three injections over six months given by a nurse and there will also be a two-year 'catch up' programme starting in 2009 to vaccinate girls under the age of 18.

The reason why under-18s only are being offered the cervical cancer vaccine is because research has shown the vaccine needs to be administered before a girl becomes sexually active. This is because the vaccines won't help prevent cervical cancer in women already infected with HPV, which can happen without you even knowing.

If girls take up the vaccination, it could well eradicate cervical cancer in around 20 years' time (the length of time it takes for HPV to cause Cervical Cancer). This means we still need the cervical screening programme in the UK, even after the vaccines become widely available, so don't forget to keep your appointment.

CHAPTER EIGHT

How to be extremely knowledgeable about sex
(without trying)

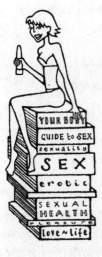

Abstinence

When you choose to abstain, i.e. not have sex for a period of time. Usually the result of realising you've been dating a hopeless case for the last six months.

AC/DC

Not a dodgy old-timers rock band, but a supposedly witty reference to someone who is bisexual, i.e. someone who fancies both boys and girls. AC/DC actually refers to electrical equipment that is adaptable for both sets of current, which is why it's also the bisexuality tag.

AIDS - *acquired immune deficiency syndrome*

A potentially fatal disease that drastically lowers the body's natural ability to fight infection and so leaves you more vulnerable to a whole host of illnesses. Transmitted via blood, vaginal secretions and semen, yet another reason why you should always practise safer sex.

Anal sex

Literally, penetrative sex in the anus as opposed to sex from behind, which is sex in the vagina but entered from behind. No longer illegal, but a good way to catch an STI, as the anus doesn't stretch which means it's prone to tearing very easily. Always ensure you use extra-strong condoms.

Aphrodisiac

A food or substance which is said to increase sexual desire, e.g. oysters and garlic. Speculative whether it works or not.

Areola

The coloured area which surrounds the nipple – it can be pink, brown or black depending on your skin tone.

Aural sex

Naughty phone sex, or talking dirty to each other. Sounds silly but actually works quite effectively if you do it right.

Balls – *testicles*

These are the two small glands found below the penis. Their role is to produce sperm and secrete the male sex hormone testosterone. Super sensitive because they are full of nerve endings. So never grab, twist or kick a guy here – unless you want him to end up in hospital.

Barrier method

Contraception that literally forms a barrier between the uterus and sperm to avoid conception taking place. Barrier methods include the condom and the cap.

Bisexual

Someone who fancies both men and women.

Blow job

Oral sex on a guy. Also known as 'giving head'. Contrary to the term, no blowing or exchange of heads is involved.

Blue balls

This is the slang name for the swelling of the testicles. It's said to occur when a boy gets aroused but doesn't ejaculate. It's called blue balls because the scrotum gets a blue tinge, though it's not dangerous and a guy can easily solve it on his own without your help.

Bondage

A consensual way of restraining your partner during sex usually using silk scarves, furry handcuffs, etc.

Boner

Slang name for an erection. A bit of a misnomer as there is no actual bone in the penis. The erection comes from blood flooding into the spongy tissues and making them rigid.

Bonking

Sex – need I say more?

Cervix

The neck of the womb, found at the back of the vagina. Highly sensitive and can be painful if it's touched during deep penetration.

Chlamydia

The most common sexually transmitted infection in the UK. Causes pelvic inflammatory disease and possible infertility if not treated.

Circumcision

The surgical removal of the foreskin, sometimes done for religious and cultural reasons or for health reasons. Has little bearing on the sensitivity of the penis.

Clap – gonorrhoea

A sexually transmitted infection, currently on the increase in the UK and cured only by seeing your doctor for powerful antibiotics.

Clitoris

The female hot spot organ – stimulation here causes arousal and orgasm. Found at the entrance to your vagina, where the two inner lips of the labia minora meet.

Coitus

Scientific term for sex.

Crabs – pubic lice

Nasty sexually transmitted critters that live and thrive in the pubic region. See your doctor, and fast, if you have them and make sure you wash all towels, bed sheets and underwear at a high temperature so you don't reinfect yourself.

Cum (pronounced come)

Also known as semen, this is a mixture of fluid and sperm and is ejected from the penis during ejaculation. It's made up of 10 per cent sperm, and 90 per cent fluids. Contrary to urban myths, during ejaculation semen doesn't shoot out like a geyser and, in fact, only a teaspoonful is released.

Cunnilingus

Oral sex on a girl. The official name for men going south.

Cystitis

Inflammation of the bladder – will feel as if you are peeing razor blades.

Deep-throating

Porn idea of oral sex, which works on the premise that a penis can penetrate a woman's throat! It can't unless you want your gag reflex to kick in and vomit to ensue.

Dildo

A penis-shaped sex toy usually made of rubber and designed for penetration.

Doggy style

Sex from a behind position (not sex in the behind).

Double-bagged

Wearing two condoms at once. A complete waste of time, because one condom will work just fine.

Douche

A vaginal rinse supposedly to help you feel cleaner down below – not recommended at it can cause infection.

Ejaculation

The emission of semen from the penis. Different to male orgasm, which is signalled by a series of involuntary contractions (though they do tend to happen at the same time).

Erogenous zones

The parts of your body that respond during sexual stimulation – look for that tingly 'Ooh' feeling.

Erotica

Books, pictures and films designed to elicit sexual arousal, though not as explicit as pornography – which usually features close-ups of genitals and sex acts.

Fantasy

An imaginary sexual scenario that you play over and over in your head and sometimes choose to act out.

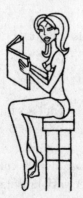

Fellatio
Blow job on a man. The official name for giving head.

Fetish
A sexual affinity to a particular body part, object or act – can be feet, shoes or even oranges!

Frigid
Supposedly a woman who is too uptight to have sex. In reality a term used by men who can't face the fact that some women don't want to have sex with them.

Foreplay
The stuff that comes before penetration – think kissing, stroking, touching and oral sex.

Foreskin
The fold of skin that covers the head of a penis. Removed when a man has been circumcised.

French kissing
Kissing with tongues.

Frenulum
Extra-sensitive ridge of skin found on the underside of the penis.

Genital warts
Sexually transmitted warts on your genitals. Caused by the HPV virus genital warts are implicated in 97 per cent of cases of cervical cancer.

Golden showers

Sexual water sports – whereby one person pees on another for sexual gratification.

G-spot

Also known as the Grafenburg spot. This is the raised hot spot on the front wall of the vagina.

Hand job

Rubbing a man's penis with your hand, until he comes.

Herpes

A sexually transmitted infection that manifests itself as small, very painful blisters. Very contagious during an outbreak.

HIV – human immunodeficiency virus

The virus that causes AIDS.

Hymen

The thin stretch of skin that covers the entrance to your vagina. Said to mark the difference between a virgin and a non-virgin. Really a load of old nonsense as the hymen can break at any time before you start having sex, through vigorous sport and with the use of tampons.

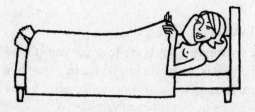

Impotence
When a man cannot get an erection and so can't have sex.

Kegels
Vaginal exercises that strengthen the PC muscles of the vagina to help you grip the penis during sex. Can be found by stopping your pee mid-flow.

Labia
Lips of the vagina. Like the lips on your face they come in all shapes and sizes.

Landing strip
This refers to women who have had most of their pubic hair waxed off and all that's left is a thin strip of hair.

Libido
Your sexual drive – that yearning you get for sex. Can be killed off with too much stress, alcohol and too little sleep.

Lubrication
KY jelly, creams and gels that add a bit of needed moisture to the genitals during sex. They can aid penetration and make sex a heck of a lot easier.

Masochist
A person who gets off on being physically hurt, spanked or slapped by someone during sex.

Masturbation
Rubbing your genital area in any way for sexual pleasure. Can be done with your clothes on or off.

Ménage à trois

A threesome – or rather a three-in-a-bed scenario.

Menstrual cycle

The 28-day cycle of your period that takes you from your monthly bleed right through to ovulation and back again.

Missionary

The most-used UK position: woman on bottom, man on top.

Mons pubis

The fleshy area above the vulva that is covered with pubic hair.

Morning-after pill

Better known as the emergency pill, as it can be taken 72 hours after unprotected sex.

Oestrogen

The female sex hormone, responsible for fertility, the menstrual cycle and female curves.

Oral sex

Stimulation of the genitals with the mouth, tongue and lips.

Orgasm

Sexual climax – look for involuntary contractions in the vagina and surrounding tissues.

Orgy

Group sex usually only viewed in porn films because who really wants to sleep with ten different men in one night?

Ovulation

The mid-monthly release of an egg from an ovary.

Penis

A shaft-shaped male organ, which on average is about 13–18cm (5–7in) when erect and 7.5cm (3in) when flaccid (despite what men would have you believe).

Perineum

The sensitive area of skin found between the front and back bottoms.

Pheromones

Secretions from the body that have no smell but supposedly stimulate instant lust in others. Artificial pheromones are now sold with dodgy-sounding names like Black Stallion.

Premature ejaculation

When a man ejaculates too soon, either as he penetrates or before penetration has taken place.

Prostate gland

A walnut-shaped gland, also known as the male G-spot, found by inserting a finger into his anal passage.

Pudenda

The proper name for women's external genitals (vulva).

Quickie

Speedy sex, usually with no foreplay or discarding of clothes.

Rimming

Oral stimulation of the anus, i.e. licking round the edge of the bottom – a good way to pick up a mouth infection.

Rubbers - condoms

Also known as Johnnies, sheaths, and French letters. The only method of contraception that protects you from HIV, STIs, and possible pregnancy.

S&M

Sadomasochism – where people willingly do bizarre things, like beat the hell out of each other, to get turned on.

Sadist

A person who 'gets off ' on inflicting pain. This usually goes hand in hand with a masochist, hence the term S&M sex.

Safer sex

Sex that carries a low risk of contracting HIV or an STI. It usually refers to limiting your sexual partners and sex with a condom.

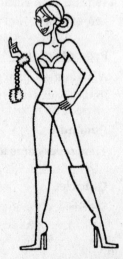

Scrotum

Pouch of skin behind the penis that contains the testicles.

Sex toys

Vibrators, handcuffs, etc.

Smegma

Cheesy, smelly stuff beneath the foreskin.

Smear test

An examination to test that the cells from the cervix are healthy and not pre-cancerous.

Sixty-nine

Simultaneous oral sex. The 69 refers to the position of your bodies while you're doing it.

Tantric sex

Trendy spiritual sex that involves holding penetration and withholding ejaculation for as long as possible.

Testosterone

The loved-up Barry White of male hormones responsible for the male sex drive, facial hair and male characteristics.

Trichomoniasis

Horrible sexually transmitted infection, which comes with a strong fishy smell and discharge.

Uncut – foreskin

The piece of skin that covers the head and glans of the penis that has not been circumcised, i.e. removed surgically.

Unprotected sex

Sex without a condom or any other form of contraception that, therefore, offers you no protection against sexual nasties and pregnancy.

Uterus

Also known as the womb.

Vagina

The spongy muscular canal that leads from the womb to the vulva. This is the area that the penis goes into during sex and a baby comes through during birth.

Vibrator

A sex toy, which is basically a penis-shaped piece of plastic with a battery inside that makes it vibrate.

Viagra

Impotence pill to help men who have trouble getting it up.

Virgin

Someone who hasn't had penetrative sex yet.

Vulva

The external female sexual organs.

Voyeur

Someone who enjoys watching people have sex or get undressed.

Wet dreams

It happens when a boy ejaculates while he is fast asleep. It's an unconscious act and is called a wet dream, because men wake up feeling, erm, wet.

Zzz... sleep

Something that happens when you're too tired after doing most of the above.

Resources

Help, advice, information and naughty shopping

UK

AVERT (Aids, Education and Research Trust)
4 Brighton Road, Horsham, West Sussex RH13 5BA
Tel: 01403 210 202 Website: www.avert.org

Breast Cancer Care Helpline Tel: 0808 800 6000

British Pregnancy Advisory Service (BPAS)
Tel: 08457 304 030 Website: www.bpas.org

Brook Advisory Young Persons Helpline
Tel: 0800 018 5023

Durex (information on condoms)
Website: www.durex.com

Family Planning Association, 50 Featherstone Street,
London EC1Y 8QU
Tel: 0845 122 8690 Website: www.fpa.org.uk

Family Planning Association (FPA), Contraceptive
Education Service Helpline
Tel: 020 7837 4044

GUM clinics in the UK call NHS Direct Tel: 0845 4647
Website: www.nhsdirect.nhs.uk

Herpes Virus Association, 41 North Road, London N7 9DP
Tel: 0845 123 2305
Website: www.herpes.org.uk

Magic Moments, 14 Rock Close, Hastings,
East Sussex TN35 4JW Tel: 01424 853 366
Website: www.adulterotica.co.uk (online suppliers for 15
years with over a million customers, they offer a secure
service with over 400 erotic products)

Marie Stopes International Tel: 0845 300 80 90
(for details of centres, abortion and contraception)
Website: www.mariestopes.org.uk

National AIDS Helpline Tel: 0800 567 123

National Childbirth Trust Information Line
Tel: 0300 3300 770

Sex Shopping Websites: www.passion8shop.com,
www.emporiolingerie.com, www.gash.co.uk and
www.blacklace-books.co.uk, www.annsummers.com

Society of Health Advisers in STDs
Website: www.shastd.org.uk

Women's National Cancer Control Campaign Helpline
Tel: 020 7729 2229
(Tues/Weds/Thurs 9.30 am to 1.00 pm)

Australia

Australian Herpes Management Forum Tel: 02 8230 3843
Website: www.ahmf.com.au

Sexual Health and Family Planning Australia
Tel: 02 6230 5255 (clinics),
Website: www.shfpa.org.au

National Breast Cancer Foundation Tel: 02 9299 4090

Sexually Transmitted Diseases Australia
Website: www.stdservices.on.net

New Zealand

Auckland Sexual Health Service Tel: 0800 739 432
Website: www.sexfiles.co.nz

Family Planning New Zealand Tel: 0800 3725463
For clinics and information go to
Website: www.fpanz.org.nz

HPV Association Tel: 0508 11 12 13
Website: www.hpv.org.nz

New Zealand Breast Cancer Foundation
Website: www.nzbcf.org.nz

South Africa

National Aids Helpline Tel: 0800 012 322
Website: www.aidshelpline.org.za

Department of Health Website: www.doh.gov.za

For the latest health news and for doctors go to:
Website: www.health24.co.za

Canada

Public Health Agency of Canada
Website: www.phac-aspc.gc.ca (list
of 550 non-profit organisations devoted to sexual
health issues)

Planned Parenthood
Tel: 613 241 4474 Website: www.ppfc.ca
(sexual and reproductive health)

USA

Planned Parenthood
Website: www.plannedparenthood.org (sexual and
reproductive health)

www.womenshealth.org – sexual health information site

www.loupaget.com – for naughty products and sex seminars

To find out more about the author: www.anitanaik.co.uk

Index

abstinence 191
AC/DC 191
'against the wall' position 104–5
AIDS 179, 192
alcohol consumption 126
anal sex 81–2, 192
anatomy 6–20
   female 6–13
   male 14–20
anti-sex brigade 53
antifungal creams 183
antioxidants 31
anus, rimming 202
aphrodisiacs 192
areola 7, 12, 192
arguments 25
arousal stage 91–2, 97–8
aural sex 192

back 47–8
'back bend', the 104
bacterial vaginosis (gardnerella)
   180–1
balconies, sex on 150–1
balls *see* testicles
barrier methods 193
   see also condoms;
diaphragm/cap
basal body temperature method
   171–2

beach, sex on 149–50
Ben Wa balls 151
benefits of sex 29–31
Billings/cervical mucus method
   171–2
bisexuals 191, 193
blood pressure 30
blow jobs (fellatio) 19, 58–63, 85,
   193, 195, 197
   champagne 148–9
blue balls 193
body, concern about your 112, 122,
123
body odour 59
body weight 28, 30, 165
boils 86
bondage 142–4, 157, 193, 202
bone strength 29
boners 193
   see also erections
boredom, sexual 29, 75–6, 121,
   122–3, 144
breast cancer 186
breast examinations 186
breasts 6–7, 12
   see also areola; nipples
bullying lovers 53–4
butt plugs 151

cancer
  breast 186
  cervical 10, 16, 185, 187–90
  testicular 16
candida albicans 182
cap/diaphragm 169–70
carcinogens 190
CAT (Coital Alignment
Technique) 99, 101–2
cervical cancer 10, 16, 185, 187–90
cervical smear test 185, 187–90, 203
cervix 10, 194
chlamydia 176–7, 194
  test 187
circumcision 15–16, 194
clap see gonorrhoea
clitoral orgasms 95
clitoris 6, 8–9, 13, 194
  and oral sex 64, 66
  sexual positions and the
    stimulation of 76–7, 78, 101–2
clothes, having sex in your 88, 105
cock rings 151
coitus 194
condoms 73, 178
  breaking 169
  double-bagged 195
  Ez-On 167
  female (Femidom) 169
  'missing' 131
  polyurethane 167
  and sex on the beach 150
  slang names for 202
  using 168
contraception 73, 160–74, 193
  barrier methods 193
  condoms 73, 131, 150, 166–9, 178,
    195, 202

contraceptive patch 173
diaphragm/cap 169–70
emergency 131, 170, 172–3, 200
female condom (Femidom) 169
implants 171
injections 171
innovations 173–4
IUD (intrauterine device) 170,
  173
IUS (intrauterine system) 170
myths regarding 161–2, 165–6,
  168–9
natural methods 171–2
percentage of women using 163
pill 162–6
and sexually transmitted
  infections 160, 162, 174, 175
smart hormones 174
vaginal microbiocides 174
vaginal ring 173–4
contraceptive patch 173
control freaks 144
crabs (public lice) 194–5
cramps, post-orgasm 132
cum 195
  see also ejaculation; semen
cunnilingus 63–5, 66–7, 110, 195
cyber sex 145
cystitis 180, 181–2, 185, 195

deep-throating 59, 195
depth of penetration 77–81, 124
DHEA (dehydroepiandrosterone)
  22, 30
diaphragm/cap 169–70
diet 30, 31
dildos 151, 195
distraction techniques 127

'doggie style' 78–9, 195
double-bagging 195
douching 184, 196
dressing up 144–5

earlobes 46
ejaculation 196
    delaying 98, 112
    female 101
    premature 41, 126–7, 201
    see also semen; sperm
emergency contraception 131, 170,
    172–3, 200
emergency pill 131, 172–3, 200
emotional stimuli 91–2, 93
endorphins 45
erectile dysfunction 86, 125–6, 199
    see also Viagra
erections 14
    hands free 99
    slang names for 193
erogenous zones 45–8, 196
    female 12–13
    male 19–20
erotica 109, 113, 137, 196
    DIY 147
Evra 173
ex-partners 118
exhibitionism 147–8
experimentation 87, 121

faithfulness, men and 27–8
faking it 41, 69–70, 101, 103, 107–8,
    113, 119
fallopian tubes 177
famous people, sex with 50, 51, 52,
    139
fantasies *see* sexual fantasies

fatigue 126
fatty acid cycle 30
feet 46
fellatio *see* blow jobs
female condom (Femidom) 169
female ejaculation 101
female genitals 7–11, 63–4, 201, 204
    external 7–9, 11, 199, 201, 204
    internal 9–10
    see also vagina
fetishism 146, 197
fidelity 27–8
fingers 46
food 30–1, 85–6, 192
    aphrodisiacs 192
    kinky sex and 148–9
forearms 48
foreplay 67–70, 91, 120, 197
foreskin 15–16, 66, 197, 203
    see also circumcision
free radicals 31
frenulum 20, 61, 197
Friday, Nancy 49
frigidity 197
fruit 148, 149
FSH (follicle-stimulating
hormone) 23

G-spot (Grafenburg spot) 6, 12, 198
    hitting 78–9, 127
    locating 84, 110
    male (prostate gland) 6, 20, 110
    and orgasm 12, 96, 102
G-spotting 102
gagging 143
gardnerella 180–1
genital herpes 178–9, 198
genital warts 177–8, 190, 197

test for 185
genitals
  female 7–10, 11, 63–4, 199, 201,
    204
  male 6, 14–20, 201, 202
  odour 63
genito-urinary infections 176,
  180–5
glans (head of the penis) 14
golden showers 198
gonorrhoea (clap) 179, 194
good sex 2–3
gossip 83
group sex 200
GUM (genito-urinary medicine)
  clinics 176
GyneFIX 170

hair 47
  see also pubic hair
hand jobs 40–1, 60–2, 65, 198
hands 46
headaches, post-orgasm 132
healthy living 31
heart disease 29, 100
herpes 178–9, 198
HIV 179, 198
home movies 147
hormones 200
  female 23–6, 109
    see also oestrogen;
    progesterone
  male 16, 21–3, 203
  smart 174
hotel balconies 150–1
human papilloma virus (HPV)
  177–8, 190, 197
  test for 185

humour 112, 133
hymen 11, 71, 72, 198

ice 85, 148–9
imagination 111, 138
immune system 100
implants (contraceptive) 171
impotence 86, 125–6, 199
  see also Viagra
infertility 177, 187
injections (contraceptive) 171
insomnia 100, 132, 204
intimacy 99
IUD (intrauterine device) 170, 173
IUS (intrauterine system) 170

Kegels 123, 199
kinky sex 135–59
  benefits 137
  bondage 142–4, 157, 193, 202
  dilemmas 155–7
  exhibitionism 147–8
  fetishism 146, 197
  hot tips 158–9
  involving food 148–9
  offensive 142, 155, 157
  outdoor 149–51
  pornography 153–4
  questions to ask about 140–2
  role-playing 144–5
  sex toys 151–2
  talking dirty 152–3, 155, 192
  threesomes 139, 157
  voyeurism 140, 147–8, 204
kissing 83, 197
knees 48
knowing what you want 111
KY jelly 120

labia majora/minora 7–8, 199
landing strip 199
lazy sex 1–2
legs 46–7
Levonelle-2 172–3
LH (luteinising hormone) 24
LHRH (luteinising hormone
releasing hormone) 22
libido *see* sex drive
location, location 116, 140, 149–51,
    156
longevity 29
love, and sex 28
lubrication 37–8, 120, 199
    for condoms 167
    flavoured 61
    for hand jobs 65
    and vaginal infections 182, 184
    and vaginal tightness 124

masochists 199
    see also S&M (sadomasochism)
massage 47–8, 113
    body-to-body 84
masturbation 32–56
    benefits 34, 37
    choosing your location 38–9
    definition 199
    making it work for you 37–8
    male 22, 39–41
    mutual 43–8
    and pornography 54–6
    positions for 38
    rules 35–9
    techniques 37
    troubleshooting tips 41–2
    turn-offs 53–4
    using vegetables 148

melatonin 31
men
    and erectile dysfunction 86,
        125–6, 199
    erogenous zones 19–20
    faking it 108
    and fidelity 27–8
    G-spot 6, 20, 110
    and masturbation 22, 39–41
    and orgasms 41–4, 63, 89–90,
        97–9, 101, 107–8
    and premature ejaculation 41,
        126–7, 201
    sex drives 21–3, 131
    sex hormones 16, 21–3, 203
    sexual anatomy 6, 14–20, 201, 202
    sexual fantasies of 52
    and sexual hygiene 16, 59
    sexual worries 125–9
    virgins 72
    see also penis
ménage à trois 139, 157, 200
menstrual cycle 11, 23–6, 200
mental stimuli 91–2, 93
    see also erotica
metabolic rate 30
mirrors 147
miscarriage 162
missionary position 71, 76–7, 111,
    128, 200
    see also plunge, the
mons pubis 7–8, 200
mood 99
morning sex 109
morning-after etiquette 133–4
morning-after pill 131, 172–3, 200
multiple orgasms 97

natural contraception 171–2
nipples 6–7, 12, 19
noisy sex 44
  see also talking dirty
NuvaRing 173–4

oestrogen 80, 200
  and bone strength 29
  of contraceptives 162, 164, 173
  hormonal cycles of 23–6
  and mood 99
  and orgasms 99
  and weight loss 30
office sex 115
oral sex 58–67, 85, 193, 200
  blow jobs 19, 58–63, 85, 148–9,
    193, 195, 197
  cunnilingus 63–5, 66–7, 110, 195
  deep-throating 59, 195
  illegal 92
  refusal 67
  sixty-nine position 64–5, 203
  trouble shooting tips 64–7
orgasm 85, 89–113
  benefits of 90, 99–100
  clitoral 95
  competitive 91
  definition 200
  duration 93, 100
  faking 41, 101, 103, 107–8, 113, 119
  and fantasies 99
  and female ejaculation 101
  G-spot 12, 102
  and hand jobs 65
  and hand-to-thigh stimulation
    47
  how to have 91–4, 109–13
  inability to reach 108

male 41–4, 63, 89–90, 97–9, 101,
    107–8
  male disinterest in your 131
  and masturbation 38, 41, 45, 106,
    113
  multiple 97
  obsession with 112
  and oral sex 63, 64, 65, 110
  physical signs of 63, 94
  refractory period 89–90
  regarding myths 100, 111
  simultaneous 97–9
  and sleep 31
  techniques 101–5
  troubleshooting tips 106–8
  types 95–9
  vaginal 96
orgies 200
outdoor sex 149–51
ovulation 164, 201
oxytocin 25, 31, 99

pain
  during sex 72, 79, 115–16, 128–9
  post-orgasm 132
painkillers, natural 45
pelvic examinations 187
pelvic inflammatory disease (PID)
  177, 179, 187, 194
pelvic-floor (PC) muscles 84, 103,
  110, 123–4, 128, 199
penis 17, 19, 201
  erections 14, 99, 193
  foreskin 15–16, 66, 197, 203
  and hand jobs 40–1, 60–2, 65, 198
  head 14
  and oral sex 60–2
  ruptured 86

size 14, 119, 127–9
penis substitutes 148
 see also dildos; vibrators
performance pressure 53–4
perineum 13, 20, 201
periods 11, 26
personal hygiene 16, 59
pheromones 201
photography, nude 148
physical exercise 22, 109
pill, the 162–6
 see also emergency pill
plateau 92–3
'plunge' position, the 104
polyurethane 167, 169
pornography 54–6, 153–4
 hardcore 153
post-sex loving 129–34
pregnancy 73, 162, 163
premature ejaculation 41, 126–7,
 201
progesterone 23–6, 162, 164
progestogen 170, 171, 173
prolonging techniques 87
prostate gland 17–18
pubic hair 7–8, 199
public lice (crabs) 194–5
public places, sex in 116, 140
pudenda *see* vulva
punishment 157

quickies 105, 124, 201

refractory period 89–90
relaxation response 100
resolution stage 94
rhythm method 171–2
rimming 202

role-playing 144–5
rough sex 184–5
rubbers see condoms

S&M (sadomasochism) 202
sadists 202
safer sex 202
same-sex sex 50, 51, 140
scary sex 117–18, 142
scrotal tug technique 87
scrotum 6, 17, 202
semen 18–19, 195, 196
 calorie content 19, 60
 and cervical smears 189
 taste 60
 see also ejaculation; sperm
sex drive (libido) 21, 199
 female 23–6, 27, 28
 maintaining 30, 34
 male 21–3, 131
 myths regarding 27, 28
 out of sync 121–2
sex education 28
sex hormones 21–6, 200
 female 23–6, 109
 male 21–3
sex laws 92, 152, 178
sex myths 1, 27–9, 51–2
 regarding contraception 161–2,
 165–6, 168–9
 regarding orgasms 100, 111
 regarding sexual fantasies 51–2
sex problems 114–34
 top female sex worries 120–5
 top male sex worries 125–9
sex toys 151–2, 155, 195, 202
sexual communication 25, 69
sexual demons 27–9

sexual fantasies 138–40, 143, 196
about famous people 50, 51, 52, 139
female 50
formation 49–50
male 52
masturbatory 36, 49–52
myths regarding 51–2
odd 51–2
same-sex 50, 51, 140
top eight 139–40
sexual health checks 185–90
sexual hygiene 16, 59
sexual positions 76–82, 101–5, 115, 195, 200
'against the wall' 104–5
CAT 99, 101–2
for large penises 128–9
missionary 71, 76–7, 111, 128, 200
'plunge' 104
'side-by-side' 80–1, 128
sixty-nine 64–5, 203
for small penises 127–8
standing up 80
and vaginal noises 121
and vaginal size 124–5
'woman on top' 77–8, 111, 124, 128–9
sexual problems 1–2
impotence 86, 125–6, 199
premature ejaculation 41, 126–7, 201
sexual questions (not to ask) 118–19
sexual statistics 87
sexually transmitted infections (STIs) 59, 73, 175–90, 192, 194, 197–8, 203
checklist 175

chlamydia 176–7, 187, 194
and contraception 160, 162, 174, 175
general symptoms 175–6
genital warts 177–8, 185, 190, 197
gonorrhoea 179, 194
herpes 178–9, 198
HIV/AIDS 179, 192
sexual health checks 185–90
trichomoniasis 180, 203
side panels 45
'side-by-side' position 80–1, 128
sixty-nine position 64–5, 203
slave fantasies 139
sleep 31, 100, 132, 204
smart hormones 174
smear tests 185, 187–90, 203
smegma 202
smoking 13, 190
speculum 187–8, 189
sperm 16, 18
spermatic cord 16
spine 47–8
spots 86
squeeze technique 127
'standing' position 80
stop/start technique 126–7
strangers, sex with 139
striptease 69
stroke 30
submission 145

talking 25
dirty 152–3, 155, 192
Tantric sex 113, 203
television 84
testicles 6, 16–17, 192
blue balls 193

testicular cancer 16
testosterone 16, 21–3, 203
in women 26
thighs 47
threesomes 139, 157, 200
thrush (candida) 180, 182–3, 184
trichomoniasis 180, 203
tummies 48
turn-offs 53–4
turn-ons 116–17
    see also erogenous zones
tying partners up 87

uncut 203
unprotected sex 203
urethra 15
urethritis 182
urinating, on your partner 198
uterus (womb) 10–11, 203

vagina 9–10, 204
    clamping up 72–3
    noise from 121
    size 123–5
vaginal cul-de-sac 88
vaginal deodorants 185
vaginal discharge 10, 175, 177, 179–82
vaginal dryness 120
vaginal microbiocides 174

vaginal orgasms 96
vaginal ring 173–4
vegetables, phallic 148
venous thromboembolism 163
Viagra 204
vibrators 151, 152, 155, 204
video cameras 147
virginity 204
    and the hymen 11, 71
    loosing 70–4
vitamin B 85
voyeurism 140, 147–8, 204
vulva (pudenda) 7–9, 201, 204

'walking out' 25
water retention 25
water sports 198
wet dreams 204
wild sex 54, 73–4, 115–18, 142
    see also kinky sex
withdrawal method 161–2
'woman on top' position 77–8, 111,
    124, 128–9
womb see uterus
wrists 48

yoghurt 183
youthfulness 30